The Lazy Lady's
Easy Diet

The Lazy Lady's
Easy Diet

A Fast-Action Plan to Lose Weight Quickly for Sustained Slenderness and Youthful Attractiveness

by
SIDNEY PETRIE
in association with
ROBERT B. STONE

PARKER PUBLISHING COMPANY, INC.

West Nyack, N.Y.

PRINTED IN THE UNITED STATES OF AMERICA

B&P

To my wife, *Iris*
and
David, Doug, Jackie, Jeff,
Lisa, Richie, and Sandy

SIDNEY PETRIE

A Foreword by a Doctor of Medicine

The pursuit of health and beauty is one of woman's most paramount concerns. As a physician and a mother I have known only too well the pitfalls in the eating habits of our modern society. I have seen how an apparently normal diet can lead to obesity as well as to malnutrition. I have seen women undertake starvation diets and other rigorous regimes only to return soon after to their former weight and having to face the problem again and again in discouragement and despair.

The authors point out these pitfalls well. They have zeroed in on the critical areas of diet. They point the accusing finger at the fat makers that prevail too prominently today. They underscore the foods that are important sources of health and beauty.

Perhaps the most valuable word in this book is "easy." By providing a technique for enjoying a permanent new way of eating, rather than going on one temporary diet after another, this book opens new doorways to sustained slenderness and youthful attractiveness.

Elizabeth Kennedy-Knuth, M.D.

What This Book Can Bring to You

Some one thousand women have played a part in the writing of this book. Their happy experiences losing weight while they gained in health and beauty under the author's care has been wrapped up for you in these pages. You can make the trip to youthful attractiveness quickly and easily, too,—so easily, so full of fun, and so free of effort, that diet acquires a whole new meaning.

Anyone can follow the simple plan in this book and see immediate results in her appearance. You can lose pound after pound during the very first week, and glow with a youthful radiance and exuberance that you may never have experienced before. Your family, friends, and acquaintances may well be astonished at the changes that are taking place in your appearance.

Most of these thousand women were referred to the author by their physicians after long and discouraging periods of unsuccessful attempts to lose weight. These attempts required effort. Many of these women deserve a medal for the herculean strength of will they exerted. But that medal would be all they would have to show for it.

On the other hand, in the author's office they found no pills, no exercising, no effort. Instead, they did find new enjoyment in eating, fascinating beauty secrets, and key nutrients for brimming over with good health and youthful vitality as they discarded unwanted pounds.

These women came over-fed or under-nourished. Within not too long a time they became slender and radiantly attractive with a glamorous new look. Furthermore, they have stayed that way according to their reports. "The Lazy Lady's Easy Diet" needs no willpower. It is a "fun" way of satisfying eating that you will want to continue. It requires minimal exercise of willpower, minimal discipline, and minimal expenditure of energy in muss and fuss over so-called diet foods.

To languish on carrot sticks, cottage cheese, and melba toast is debilitating to the body and soul. It is rejuvenating to the body and soul to enjoy eating such epicurean foods as veal parmesan or chicken luau, without misgivings and worries as to the possibilities of gaining unwanted pounds.

You can eat satisfying foods and still lose weight fast! At the same time, using nature's own nutrients, you can build your body's youth and beauty to amazingly high levels. And no hard, harsh discipline is required. Everything you need to know and use in your own home is here in this book—complete calorie tables, the mineral and vitamin foods, menus galore, scores of delicious recipes, and a step-by-step procedure that spells fun in securing and keeping a glamorously trim figure. Recognizing that we all are lazy—if there's an easier way to do something we all want to know that way—this book provides dieters with the path of least resistance.

Pounds of excess weight permanently off your body, years of unwanted aging off your appearance, renewed youthful glamour—this is a big promise for a book to make! Yet it is a promise fulfilled for a thousand women and now with the help of this book, it can begin to come true for you just as fast as you want it to happen. It's easy. Try it. You'll see for yourself and you'll like what you see.

Sidney Petrie

Contents

The Lazy Lady's
Easy Diet

1

The Key to Effortless Weight Reduction
for Youth and Beauty

Some women stay thin effortlessly. Others diet and diet and diet on an endless and agonizing cycle of weight loss and weight gain. Which type are you?

Psychologists know that the only way people can stay slim permanently is effortlessly, because as soon as effort is involved, failure is on the way! In fact, they know that the harder you try, the sooner you fail.

It follows that only an easy diet can really succeed. Find a way of pleasurable eating that knocks the pounds off you without an ounce of effort, and you have it made.

A Diet That Does Not Require Will Power

Impossible, you say; all diets require will power. Nonsense, I say; and I have 1,000 women to back me up. These are the women who have been referred to me by their physicians, family or friends and who have lost weight easily. And remember, easily means permanently, where losing weight is concerned. My overweight clients leave thin and never come back.

How many times have you lost the battle royal between conscience and garlic bread, or between will power and rissole potatoes? Give up; you always will.

Many more fat people eat melba toast than thin people, not because they like it, but because it's thin like they want themselves to be. Yet, fat they regain and fat they remain. Little do they know

1

they would be better off eating something they enjoyed, even if it were a thick slice of imported cheese. That enjoyment, plus some of the secrets about food on the pages ahead, would make them thin.

Eat What You Like—But

Madame Herve Alphand, wife of the former French ambassador to Washington and one of the most chic and elegant women in Paris, calls her painless way of keeping slim a "no-diet" plan. She eats everything she likes, but in modest quantities. She is in the habit of never eating too much or drinking too much. To her, it's as "easy as pie."

Her plan is good. *It's good because it works for her.* However, it *may not work for you.* It may be easy for her to be satisfied with one portion of crepe suzettes. But those French pancakes may be irresistible to you and you have to have three portions or die trying. Enjoy yourself when you eat. Change anything else when you diet, but don't change that.

What the "Easy Diet" Is

One thousand women, a total of 30,000 pounds lighter—permanently pounds lighter. I'd judge they looked a total of 10,000 years younger, and somewhere there are 1,000 interested men who would probably back me up on that.

Do I reach into a file and give them a typewritten menu? Do I dispense appetite-killing pills? Do I prescribe exercises? Not at all!

And there are no steam rooms or vibrators in my office. No pounding, pressing, pinching. No fads or fasting. Just information, instructions and advice. Oh, yes, there is one other activity that does take place, but I'd prefer to divulge that later.

What then is this easy diet? If I were to try to summarize what it is, I would say that it is a nutritious diet designed to fit each woman's present eating habits.

Since each woman's eating habits are different, the easy diet is different for each woman. This book will tell you how to create the easy diet for yourself, built on nutritional truths you will discover, and designed to fit your present eating habits.

The 1,000 Women I Helped Grow Thin Effortlessy

I will tell you about these women—the social "outcast" who lost 80 pounds and regained her friends, the hefty ex-model who was able to return to modeling, the 750-pound foursome of sisters who lost a collective 250 pounds, the young married girl who saved her marriage, the many who won back their youth, health, and beauty.

These are the 1,000 women whose clinical weight loss records average 30 pounds each in less than six months each, and no weight return.

The Case of a 38-Year-Old Mother "on and off" Diets All Her Life

Madeleine B. is typical. A thirty-eight-year-old mother of two teenage boys, she weighed 185 when she came to me at the suggestion of her physician. She had been on and off diets what she said seemed to be during "all my life." She said she figured she had already lost and regained twice her current weight. She had been as low as 125 in the last ten years and as high as 195, hitting the tops and bottoms a number of times. Her husband, a pilot with a large airline, urged her to seek medical help, but diet pills gave her skin problems and made her feel continuously listless.

I made Madeleine keep track of what she ate, and when she ate, for one week. When she returned with her chart, we went over her eating habits. Here is what we found. She ate hardly any breakfast and only a very light lunch. She liked an afternoon coffee break, ate a normally large dinner, and wound up the evening with an icebox snack. I saw an occasional coke and beer along the way, but by and large, that was it.

Madeleine and I then agreed on certain changes. The times for her meals and snacks would remain basically the same, but we'd make some trades or substitutions: eggs or bacon instead of toasted muffin, a hamburger steak for a hamburger sandwich, a second vegetable for potatoes. There were a few others, but nothing crucial. Madeleine gave me a patronizing look when she left. She was obviously expecting no miracles.

A week later she returned. The scale showed she had lost two pounds. "It's going to be a long pull, at this rate," she said. "Any hunger pangs or battles with temptation?" I asked. She confessed it was so easy she really had not expected to lose at all. "Well, then," I reminded her, "What difference does time make!" We made only a few more changes that visit in her eating routine and habits.

Madeleine checked in with me again about a month later. She had lost ten pounds and was feeling fine. I checked her eating habits over the last three days. She was right on target. She claimed that she was eating better than ever, had become interested in high-protein cookery, and her family was happy about the whole deal.

End of the story: Six months later Madeleine weighed 132. She was no longer losing, nor was she gaining. She had not been depriving herself of anything, so there was no regimen or diet to stop. I never saw her again. It's been over two years now. A bridge club friend of hers, age forty-four, weight 168, tells me she looks great!

My Clients' Former Diet Experiences Follow a Common Pattern

All the women in my office life—whether motion picture stars or secretaries—have one common denominator: in the past they have been unsuccessful in following diets for any length of time; they have not reacted to diets they followed; or, they have gained back all the weight they lost when they stopped dieting.

Those who have not stayed on a diet any length of time were obviously depriving themselves of an important factor in their life—the *enjoyment of food.* Those who did not react to the diet they followed were the victims of carbohydrates—the culprit among foods that can manufacture excess pounds on 1,000-calorie diets. Those who gained back all the weight they lost once they stopped dieting have some bad habits to change—like escaping from their troubles in a box of chocolate.

> LESSON: *Enjoy an easy diet, limit intake of carbohydrate foods, and learn an effortless way to change eating habits. That is what 1,000 women learned from me and that is what this book is all about.*

The Voice of Hunger and Its Myths

There is no call louder than that of the empty stomach. That call has made history through the ages. It has started wars, created new countries, brought rulers to power, and caused their downfall.

The diet that brings hunger with it might just as well end now! It must fail. No encouraging words will do. They are drowned in the din of hunger's call. Not one of my 1,000 women have ever experienced the kind of prolonged hours of hunger that the starvation diets so common among diet specialists bring about. I'd rather they have a small steak or a few pieces of chicken to tide them over. There are no hunger pangs in this book.

It is not always more food that stops hunger. Hunger's voice is heard not only when the stomach is empty, but also when the body is mineral-starved or lacking in some essential nutrient. In fact, poverty and underproduction in the world's developing countries are due largely to hungry people who cannot do a day's work because they are hungry, people who do not eat the *right kinds of food* in the right proportion. Another bowl of rice fails to satisfy hunger, when the voice of hunger is calling for nutrients needed to build muscles, blood and other blood tissues.

At a recent Far Eastern Symposium on Nutrition held in Manila, the Philippine Secretary of Health told how children are dying early in life, and how men and women become invalids in what should be the prime of life, all because of their body's hunger for nutrients to protect teeth, eyes, skin and bones. In Vietnam, the Nutrition Laboratory has research under way on the development of nutritional standards for the nutrient-starved people there. Diet deficiency has brought appalling tooth decay. Nutritional improvement is needed most acutely by Vietnamese children whose bodies are growing.

Good nutrition in this country of ours is easy to come by. It is there for the eating. It takes no pull with the local politicians, just know-how, to give the body's cells the quantity and quality of nourishment they require.

Doctors at the Mayo Brothers' famous clinic in Rochester, Minnesota, are finding that a vast number of ailments can be cured by correcting a diet deficiency. What is more, by balancing nutrition they are able to arrest body deterioration and literally prolong life.

The body needs natural food vitamins and minerals to keep the voice of hunger stilled and the body in proper repair. My 1,000 women understand the A, B, C, D, and E of vitamins. They know Vitamin A beautifies the eyes and the skin, the importance of Vitamin B to the nerves and heart, of C to resistance to disease, of D and E to strong bones and vitality.

Dieting is made easier by including the foods that keep the body well supplied with these vitamins and the voice of hunger stilled.

Did you know that iodine aids the thyroid gland to maintain a healthy metabolic rate, which in turn burns off excessive fat? Did you know that calcium is needed by mature adults just as essentially as children to provide hardness to teeth and bones? Did you know that minerals generally help to maintain body fluids and keep them from becoming too acid or too alkaline?

How can one possibly get all of the necessary vitamins, minerals, and proteins into a semi-starvation, 1,000-calorie-a-day diet? The answer is you cannot. And the sooner you realize this, the sooner you will quit tormenting your body with these famines and get on a fuller, zestier way of eating that may lose you less weight per day but lose you more weight in the long run.

How to Answer the Call of Youth by Balanced Nutrition, Not Food Fads

Supply your body with all the nutrients you need in moderation and you can have the look of youth and beauty in face and body, even beyond sixty. You can be sexually active and vital beyond seventy. You can end serious health problems that you have come to accept—hypertension, fatigue, high blood pressure, indigestion, etc.

Excess Fat Is a Killer

I hope to lead you in this book to the new vitality and strength of dynamic youth. I want you to tap new strength, new energy, and new endurance. I want you to make people gasp when you tell them your age—if you dare.

Why is it that insurance companies raise the premium rate for overweight clients? Why is it that many jobs are not open to over-weight people, and that surgeons often advise against an operation if a patient is excessively rotund. It may be hard to face up to, but excess fat will usually become your pallbearer.

Fat kills women who would otherwise be healthy, beautiful and long-lived. It cuts them down much too soon just as sure as they're born. Insurance men can tell you as a mathematical fact just how many years off your life ten excess pounds will take. The longer you carry the ten pounds, the surer you are of living up to the statistical prediction and shortening your life expectancy. Take off pounds and you add healthy years to your life.

According to life insurance statistics a thirty-five- to forty-five-year-old woman who is up to 25 percent overweight (up to 30 or 40 pounds) will die seven years sooner. If she takes off those extra pounds she will be able to live out her birthright of seventy-seven years (at least).

If you are up to 60 percent overweight, things can get pretty sticky. The longevity table says that at forty years of age, a woman has every right to expect to live to seventy-seven. However, if she weighs 208, instead of her proper 130 (at height 5'1"), and does not take it off, she may not live to see fifty-five.

What will kill her? The facts of life and death show that a prolonged state of overweight invites cardiovascular and renal diseases. These are problems of the heart, blood vessels and kidneys. It also invites pains of the bones and joints, malfunctioning of the digestive system, overtiredness and persistent fatigue. Seriously overweight women are often chronically ill with a number of health problems. Doctors estimate that overweight can increase the death rate by 50 percent for heart patients, 75 percent for kidney disease patients, and even a greater percentage for diabetics.

Doctors will tell you that on the menu for the seriously overweight are: *arthritis,* with its incurable pain; *diabetes,* a metabolic disorder in which the body's ability to oxidize (burn up) carbohydrates is hampered; *inflammation of the gall bladder; coronary thrombosis,* the medical term for a common form of heart disease; *high blood pressure, cirrhosis of the liver, etc.* There is really no end to the health problems for the obese person, except that morbid one spelled out in the insurance mortality tables.

To compound the risks, many problems that are curable by surgery for average weight people offer serious risks to the overweight. Operations for the removal of the appendix or gall bladder are fatal four times as often. Ask the nearest surgeon. A famous popular singing star of large girth had to lose 60 pounds before her physician would approve a necessary operation for gall stones.

And that's not all. Overweight women are prone to accidents due to their lessened agility, and slower reflexes. Fertility goes down as weight goes up. Overweight women becoming pregnant are candidates for complications in pregnancy, and have a greater chance of a stillborn child.

The Real Answer—Stop "Dieting"

Had enough? Then the answer is not to start dieting, but to *stop dieting.* Where has starvation gotten you? The answer is to start eating correctly, instead of starving yourself. Go on the easy, eatwell diet to look young, stay well, become more beautiful and live longer.

The enjoyable changes in your eating habits which you will soon make are easy to make and are changes for the better, not only better health and appearance, but better eating. Hormones are fine, but they make a tasteless, poor repast alongside a delicious broiled steak and crisp salad. Food supplements and health tonics are fine, but why not enjoy the tang of a grapefruit; why not savor the tantalizing flavor of freshly broiled swordfish, or of properly aged camembert.

Beware of Quickie Drug Gimmicks

Congressional investigators and the California Medical Association are taking a long, hard look at physicians who specialize in obesity by handing out drugs which reduce weight but which cause ailments that other doctors must then treat. One Beverly Hills internist who is making an effort to investigate these activities has accused these weight-control specialists of giving their patients drugs which lead to heart trouble and may even cause cancer. These drugs include amphetamines, originally developed to help war-time pilots fight off sleep; digitalis, which slows down heart action, and thyroid extracts which speed it up; and pituitary extracts which are suspected to be cancerogenic.

There will always be new "youth-giving injections," but good food will go on forever. I remember a decade or two ago a Rumanian scientist came up with an injection of serum that was the rage, but has long since faded from view. Now I see where another discovery has been made in Rumania. A biochemist there claims to have developed a "youth cocktail" that reverses some of the chemical effects of aging. A potion containing the amino acid cysteine increases the body's sulphur-hydrogen molecules which are said to decline with older age. The result is a diminishing of some visible effects of aging. Great! But I'll still bet on the goodness of vital nutrients of fresh food in the long run. And my 1,000 young-looking women bet with me—if they are not busy enjoying a martini or munching butterfly shrimp.

Beauty an Inside Job

We are what we eat, yes, but we are more than that. We are what we think and feel. Often what we think and feel affects what we eat. The lovely Judy Garland's weight has fluctuated with the intensity of the problems in her life.

Some Scottish doctors reduce very fat people by giving them no food at all, just tea, coffee and vitamin pills. Can you guess what happens when a woman who has lost 100 pounds in nine months goes back to her regular life. You're so right. In the same kitchen of the same house with the same boredom, the same routine, the same personality conflicts—food returns as her only escape from "reality."

She Ate When She Was Depressed

"When I get depressed, I wind up in the kitchen for something to eat," a young mother told me. It so happens her husband worked on the night shift and moonlighted a second income on weekends. When she wanted to chat with him, he was either sleeping or at work. She felt frustrated, alone and bored. Obviously, a change in eating habits could only be triggered by a change in living habits. I encouraged her to have a down-to-earth talk with her husband. Two incomes are not better than one if the expense is a loss of mutual happiness. It turned out that it was extremely difficult for him to change his work habits, but once this was done her overeating habits were more easily replaced with a normal routine.

The emotions, attitudes and feelings that cause women to overeat are almost too numerous to identify. Depression, boredom, and frustration joined by hostility, insecurity and fear, are leading contenders as major motivators.

It so happens that these emotions show on the face and in the posture, too. A girl with worries acquires a haggard look of a woman twice her age. Women with heavy problems walk stooped over as if the weight of the world was on their shoulders. Thus do emotions rob us of our good looks, while at the same time bringing about physiological imbalances internally that sooner or later spell disease.

I remind my clients that *weight* problems often result from *weighty* problems. It might be that once they recognize this fact they can do something intelligent about it.

Obesity, an Element of One's Self-Image

I recognize similar personality traits in overweight women. Yet, everybody is different and nobody can write a book to take the place of the psychiatrist. In some cases, even dieting and losing weight can pose a serious emotional problem that requires professional assistance; obesity can have become an important part of a person's self-image and play a vital role in interpersonal relationships. For such a person, the loss of weight can become tantamount to loss of identity, and may threaten his or her very adaptation to life. For instance, obesity caused by a subconscious need to dominate other people can become a vital factor in life with loss of weight creating a serious psychiatric problem.

But most emotions and attitudes can be controlled by the individual once recognized for what they are. Often they are the instigators of that second helping of dessert, that box of chocolate, those extra coffee breaks, or just plain gluttony.

I was sitting at a lunch counter one day. The thoughtful counterman greeted his regulars like he was dispensing slippers and cold compresses, "Your Mom give you a hard time last night, Ellen?" he asked, setting out an extra large slice of apple pie à la extra large mode. "The boss at it again today, Doris?" he coos; "We got bread pudding." The way I helped many of my 1,000 women to help themselves can possibly help you and you may find clues to your own personality on the pages ahead.

Looking at the positive side, even the problem-less individual, if she exists, can improve herself psycho-dynamically. She can face the moment with more enthusiasm and optimism. She can relate to people with more respect and understanding. She can go about her activities with more self-assurance and self-appreciation. All of this is radiated to others. It is an attractiveness and a vitality that are important contributors to beauty.

So what? You cannot just turn these things on. That's true. But they do come easier with a well-nourished mind and body. They do come easier with a loss in weight, and they do come easier with a simple self-improvement program of reconditioning. They will come to you as you follow the programs in this book.

How To Enjoy Life While You Lose Weight

The austere life that carrot sticks and melba toast symbolize is one we can stand for so long, but then we start counting the days when we can enjoy life again. It has been estimated that a strongly motivated dieter can stay on a reducing diet for about two months comfortably. The same sources admit that a balanced maintenance diet can be adhered to indefinitely.

I consider the enjoyment of food to be a necessary part of reducing and maintenance diets alike. I cannot say that I understand the psychological reasons behind this as well as psychologists do, but I am as sure of it as I can be. My clients testify to this fact.

Support of this belief sometimes comes from unexpected directions. A study of married women recently reported on at an annual meeting of the Eastern Psychological Association discloses that women who enjoy food the most are also able to enjoy sex more fully. One researcher said that the best predictors of a woman's being able to enjoy a sex life is her ability to enjoy food. The general attitude toward food was included in the study because, like sexuality, it has a clear object and involves a definite body response at the time of gratification. The correlation was called positive and significant.

I promise nobody a better sex life. But I do promise beauty and attractiveness as you grow permanently slimmer the easy diet way. And there is the promise of better health that comes with normal weight. Fulfillment of these promises are just pages away.

One promise I want you to start realizing now. It is the promise of youth. You can begin right now to pave the way for a younger look by understanding and believing that it can come about. If you refuse to believe that providing your body with nutrients it may not have been receiving can revitalize your body's tissues, you can actually stave off the new look of youth.

The body responds to belief in an amazing fashion. Suggestion can trigger illness or health. What happens in a plane when one passenger becomes sick? Others follow who may have never been airsick before. What happens on a parade field when one soldier faints? Get some more stretchers ready. What happens when a person with rose fever walks into a room with artificial plastic roses? Pass the tissues please!

Turn it around the other way. What happens to a person who cannot swim but in the process of learning realizes she can? She does swim well enough! What happens to a person who receives a "sugar pill" (placebo) from a doctor who cannot find anything organically wrong? Usually she gets well. What happens to a woman who used to think that old age was inevitable and finds out that its inevitability is still decades away? She permits herself to look young.

Permit yourself to accept youth and beauty now. Visualize yourself the fine-looking attractive woman that you really are. Visualize yourself as naturally thin, pleasingly slender. Visualize your true self as a vital, popular, and effective person.

You have started a very important transformation through your power of visualization, acceptance and belief. Don't think any less of this truth because it has been such an easy first step to take. Watch the pounds melt away and the vision comes true just a few more easy steps away.

Review of Chapter Highlights

You do not have to be on a strict diet to lose weight. You lose more weight in the long run on a nourishing regime high in protein, vitamins, and minerals. When you take weight off you add years to your life span. When you enjoy a diet, you stay slender permanently.

2

How To Lose Unwanted Pounds and
Win Your Beauty Birthright

Let's get down to business—the business of losing weight easily and staying thin and svelte *without dieting*. In the past, getting down to business in losing weight has always meant counting calories. Calories will still count, but you won't have to count them.

Counting calories has always been too difficult for anyone to do effectively and accurately. Nobody can be ultra-sure. No two portions are ever exactly alike. Recipes differ. Chefs in restaurants have their secret ingredients. Memories slip. Amateur mathematicians err.

A 1,000-calorie "intention" can prove out at 1,500 calories with just a sliver of pie that "didn't really count" and two glasses of beer at midnight ("It's too late to count it on today's and too early to begin tomorrow's").

Many women tell me that they gain weight on 1,000 calories— honest count. I believe them. But I also believe that they do not count that stick of gum every hour or that hard candy or that soft drink or that nibble that is "hardly worth figuring."

How To Gain or Lose Weight on 1,000 Calories Daily Intake

There is one way to gain weight on 1,000 calories a day or slightly over: Make those calories all carbohydrates; breakfasts of doughnuts or danish; lunches of pizza or pie; and dinners of spaghetti or other starches. You won't have to wonder very long about how much

13

you'll take off. Just eat away and watch the scales take off to show you "pounds plus."

There is one sure way to lose weight on 1,000 calories a day or even more: Include in those calories a minimum of carbohydrates; breakfasts of eggs sunnyside up and bacon; lunches of hamburger steak and salad, dinners of roast chicken and vegetable. You will lose weight; no doubt about it.

What To Do First To Control Weight

Obviously, the first order of business is learning to recognize carbohydrates so they can be avoided wherever possible. Before you are finished with this chapter you will be able to tell carbohydrate foods from proteins and fats. You will begin to recognize them for the fattening culprits that they are.

The Carbohydrate Menace to Your Normal Weight

We live in a carbohydrate age. Carbohydrate foods are easily pre-packaged and quickly prepared. They are ideal foods for mass distribution and for busy people on the run. The supermarkets would be half bare without them. Can you imagine what your local store would look like without shelves of dry cereals, a bread and cake department, that whole aisle of crackers and cookies, macaroni products, potatoes, flour and bake mixes, rice, candy and nuts, soda, sugar and freezers of ice cream?

Fifty years ago things were different. Oh, people ate cereal for breakfast, or pancakes, but it was far more common to see what we today call a country breakfast: sausages, bacon, eggs, cheese. Bread was made at home and when the loaf was gone there was no fresh box of crackers to open and Mom had the cookies well hidden. Italian pastas were yet to flood our shores and ice cream was still a novelty. No instant puddings, dehydrated potatoes, store-made pies. The sandwich was just beginning to gain in popularity. And generally, people were thinner. Are you beginning to get the message? *The first order of business for you now is to divide foods into two camps.* The *high* carbohydrates, and the *low* carbohydrates. You will protect yourself from one camp, and enjoy yourself in the other. Next order of business will be to recognize which of the low carbohydrate foods are rich in the nutrients your body needs for health and beauty. *Since you can eat more on this regimen, you can literally eat your way to both more health and more beauty,* and that includes your trim figure.

There will be further business on the agenda—the business of using clothes and cosmetics to make you look your slender best (tips I learned working with models and actresses). Then there's the business of tailoring your *attitudes* to rid your *emotions* of fat-causing frustrations and tensions. The business of using suggestion to reprogram your habits with effortless control through a process known as auto-conditioning. These and others pave the easy road ahead to the slender, vibrant, beautiful *you*. But we are getting ahead of ourselves. Back to the carbohydrates and that most important first step for your future happiness of youth, health, and beauty.

What Is a Carbohydrate?

To you and me a carbohydrate is sugar or starch which the body uses as a hook on which to hang its fat. The dictionary has a somewhat more scientific type of definition, using such words as "compounds," "cellulose," "metabolism." A simplified dictionary version might be: "a food such as sugar and starch used by plants and animals in their chemical processes."

The best this definition does for us is to clear up any misconception that a carbohydrate is some kind of strange substance that you very seldom come across. It would be very fortunate for us indeed, if this were true. If we would stumble over only the minimum carbohydrate our body needs for its chemical processes, we would all be thinner and longer lived.

No, rather it's a very common substance and in its almost pure state can take many forms: a hard white substance we bake and boil called a potato; a loaf of soft material which we slice and call bread; tiny white granules we call sugar.

Because it takes many forms, it is taken or eaten in many forms: Corn is 68 percent carbohydrate, honey is 80 percent, chestnuts are 78 percent. Apple pie is 42 percent carbohydrate; a peanut butter sandwich is 31 percent carbohydrate, a Chinese egg roll is 33 percent carbohydrate. Orange juice is practically 100 percent carbohydrate.

How To Watch for the Carbohydrate Warning Flag

The higher the percentage of carbohydrate, the bigger and redder the warning flag regarding your weight control. *The average carbohydrate percentage of a food that is safe to keep you thin is 15 percent.* You can forget those 1,000-calorie starvation diets, if you can keep your carbohydrate intake average in foods to 15 percent or below. Eat 2,000 calories and even more and you will not be likely to gain weight at a 15 percent carbohydrate level.

Does this mean you cannot eat anything with 16 percent carbohydrate or more? Of course you can! Have yourself a teaspoon of sugar if you absolutely must. But then bring your average down the rest of the day with the glorious, tempting, nourishing parade of foods that have less than 3 percent carbohydrate and even zero percent carbohydrate. Enjoy a steak smothered in sautéed mushrooms. Then, how about a glass of dry champagne as a toast to your new loveliness? Would you like roquefort cheese dressing on your salad? Beef, pork, veal, poultry, fish, cheese, eggs—there are hundreds of ways of preparing these zero to 3 percent foods that can keep you in new, interesting and varied menus for years.

To repeat, remember you can *average* as high as 15 percent. On a 2,000-calorie day most people can have 300 calories of carbohydrate foods and still not budge the scale upward. This embraces fruits and vegetables and still more delicious recipes for your new eating ways. It embraces the kind of mineral- and vitamin-packed foods that rejuvenate your tissues and revitalize your body.

It does not embrace the high carbohydrate foods. They can quickly account for 300 carbohydrate calories. (A danish in the morning and a piece of apple pie at night and you've had it for carbohydrates.) To use up your carbohydrate quota this way is to deprive yourself of those healthful foods that have medium carbohydrate count as well as high beauty count.

Most dieters are calorie counters. I don't call it easy dieting when you have to count calories. I don't propose that you count calories. I am not even going to tell you what a calorie is. If you don't know, you are better off! You will have an easier time getting thin and beautiful not counting them. I don't want you to average, or to figure percentages either. I'm going to make it real easy as follows:

How To Recognize Low Carbohydrate Foods

In Table 1 are lists of foods. They are the foods that you can eat your fill of and satisfy your hunger. You won't be as tempted to overeat when you eat abundantly of these foods, because they are the nourishing foods that satisfy hunger more fully. They also satisfy your need to enjoy the food you eat. No bland melba toast, carrot sticks and lettuce restrictions on this bill of fare; but rather it is broiled mackerel, Swedish meatballs, cheeseburgers, barbequed chicken and frankfurters, and if your tastes are more expensive—coq au vin, filet mignon, and pheasant under glass. Easy? I'll say that you will say—"It most surely is easy!"

Lists Make It Easy

The foods on these lists run from zero to 30 percent carbohydrates. A rule through the list indicates the 15 percent mark. Foods above the rule are less than 15 percent carbohydrate; foods below the rule are more than 15 percent carbohydrate. But in no case are they greater than 30 percent. This means that if you eat as many foods above the rule as you do below the rule you are generally going to average your 15 percent intake of carbohydrates or less. To make it even easier, if you eat these foods at random, you will average below 15 percent because there are more than twice as many foods listed above the rule as below!

You don't see any cereal, bread, cookies, crackers, cakes or other flour items on this list. Missing also are macaroni products and sandwiches. Desserts do not include pies, sweets or ices.

You do see meats and vegetables, fruits and salads. There are gravies, sauces and dressings. Fish, poultry, eggs and cheeses are in abundance. There is a choice of beverages, hot and cold, alcoholic and non-alcoholic.

One forty-eight-year-old real estate agent, who was having a hard job lugging her 190 pounds around the houses she was showing clients, took one look at these lists and said, "You must be kidding. I came here to lose weight, not to gain it." I explained some of the "fats of life" to her. Two weeks later she had eaten her weight down seven pounds.

Let me repeat some points to remember about this list:

1. You can eat all you want of those foods above the line.

2. You will be satisfied with less.

3. Eat at least as many of the items above the line as you do below.

4. Balance your menu by list hopping—some from here, some from there.

5. Avoid foods that are not on the list.

Table 1

LOW CARBOHYDRATE FOODS

(Eat All You Want Above Rules for That Division of Foods)

MEATS

Steak
Roast beef
Pot roast
London broil
Chopped steak
Brisket
All other cuts of beef
Sweetbreads
Tongue
Lamb chops
Leg of lamb
All cuts of lamb
Pork chops
Salt pork
Pork shoulder
Roast loin of pork
Fresh ham
Smoked ham
Bacon
All other cuts of pork
Veal chops
Roast veal
All other cuts of veal
Bologna
Frankfurters
Sausage
Salami
Kidneys (all types)
Liver (all types)
Corned beef hash
Dried beef

Round steak, swiss
Meat pie

CHEESE

American
Camembert
Münster
Cream
Limburger
Liederkranz
Swiss
Roquefort
Cheddar
Gruyère
Gorgonzola
Gouda
Fondue

Welsh rarebit

SOUPS

Bouillon
Consommé
Chicken
Julienne
Clam bisque
Lobster bisque
Cream of mushroom
Cream of asparagus
Cream of celery
Cream of spinach
Cream of tomato
Oyster stew

Pea
Lentil

VEGETABLES

Mushrooms
Soybeans
Chinese cabbage
Cucumber
Taro shoots
Lettuce
Romaine
Olives
Spinach
String beans
Celery
Tomatoes
Escarole
Mustard greens
Turnips
Cauliflower
Cabbage
Broccoli
Kale
Okra
Dandelion greens

Carrots
Squash
Beets
Peas
Artichokes

MEAT EXTENDERS

Tomato, cheese, rarebits
Chop suey
Chow mein
Tamale pie

Spanish rice
Enchilada
Chili con carne

SAUCES

Mushroom
Hollandaise
Butter
Tartar
Cheese
Curry
Tomato

SAUCES (*cont.*)

White
Egg
Cream
Soy
Mint

Orange
Vanilla
Lemon
Brown sugar

SALAD DRESSING

Roquefort
Mayonnaise
French
Thousand Island

Russian

CEREALS (cooked)

Creamed wheat
Oatmeal
Farina
Cornmeal

Rice, white
Rice, wild
Rice, brown

BREAD

Popovers

CRACKERS

Soybean (cocktail)

DESSERTS

Custard
Gelatin
Whipped cream
Rice pudding
Tapioca pudding

Cornstarch pudding
Fresh Coconut pudding

Macadamia nuts
Brazil nuts
Walnuts
Custard pie
Pumpkin pie
Squash pie
Ice cream
(See fruits)

BEVERAGES

(Non-alcoholic)
Coffee (no sugar)
Tea (no sugar)
Sauerkraut juice
Postum
Tomato juice
Buttermilk
Ovaltine

Limeade
Lemonade
Milk

BEVERAGES

(Alcoholic)
Martini
Scotch
Bourbon
Rye
Gin
Rum
Brandy
Red wine
Vermouth
Champagne, dry
Sherry dry

Highball
Sours
Punch

POULTRY

Chicken
Pheasant
Turkey
Duck
Goose
Guinea hen
Squab
Chicken liver
Creamed chicken
Pâté de foie gras

Croquettes

FISH

All types
Canned
Fresh
Smoked
Salted
Anchovies
Lobster
Crabs
Mussels
Clams
Sardines
Scallops
Oysters

FLOUR

Soybean

EGGS

All types
(cooked any way)

FATS

Corn oil
Crisco
Mineral oil
Suet
Bacon fat
Meat drippings

FATS (*cont.*)

Lard	Buttermilk	Watermelon
Olive oil	Sour cream	
Peanut oil		Oranges
Fish oil	Sweet cream	Pears
Butter	Milk	Pineapple
Oleomargarine		Cherries, sour
Whipped cream	FRUITS	Grapes
Cream	Rhubarb	Honeydew melon
	Cantaloupe	Fruit juices
Peanut butter	Strawberries	Apples
	Avocado	Banana
MILK PRODUCTS	Peaches	(Canned fruits
Yogurt	Plums	only if water
Whipped cream	Grapefruit	packed.)

Welcome to the World of Protein

Fantastic, isn't it? Do you believe you can lose weight eating all you want of this vast scope of delicious foods? You will soon prove it to yourself, and you will kiss your goodbye forever to those *dreary diet days you once knew.*

Let me just remind you once more of the foods that are not on the list. THERE IS NO BREAD. This means hamburgers and cheeseburgers served on a plate *without a bun.* THERE ARE NO POTATOES. If "french fries" are a favorite of yours, forget them. Think of something better in their place. (How about french fried onion rings!) Avoid corn, go easy on rice. Remember all that cottage cheese you ate on diets? Some of it may be still with you as fat. It's reasonably high in carbohydrate calories (27 percent).

A number of desserts are taboo for you now. You would not dream of eating those rich, gooey sundaes, or iced cake. Instead, you will be devoting your appetite to more of the lusty foods and ending up with a light dessert.

At the bar, beer is out (unless it's that new low carbohydrate type). Drink liquor without sweet mixers. Ask for your rye, scotch or vodka on the rocks, or with water. Dry wines are fine for weight control, sweet wines are definitely out. At the soda fountain, make it lemonade, iced tea or iced coffee, never regular soda pop. The diet, sugar-free kind is all right, but I am not placing the so-called low-calorie soda on your list. There is still some doubt as to whether it should be consumed on a regular or indiscriminate basis. Long-range aftereffects are a distinct possibility. That is why the label on the bottles, cartons and cans of sugar-free diet foods *warn that it should be used only by persons who wish to restrict their sugar intake,* diabetics, etc.

What Proteins Are and How They Are Used by the Body

Most of the foods on these lists are proteins. A dictionary definition of protein, boiled down to simple terms, is "organic compounds occurring naturally in all living matter and forming an essential part of animal food requirements." The word derives from the Greek "proteios" meaning primary, or holding first position, and that is exactly where they belong in every person's diet.

Proteins are body builders and repairers. Muscles, skin, hair, nails and internal organs depend on continuous supplies of new protein to retain their strength, vitality, and beauty.

All of the foods on the list are either high in fats or proteins. The high protein foods are the meat, poultry, fish and eggs. Fish is about 100 percent protein and is therefore a wonderful food to create a liking for.

Fish protein concentrate is now being used to combat malnutrition among underprivileged people throughout the world. In Korea, it is being used as an additive to their present carbohydrate-heavy foods. The concentrate was originally introduced by an Illinois firm, but the Koreans are now building their own plant to manufacture it.

Ever hear of shark-eating men? Both shark and whale meat are considered delicacies in Iceland, where fresh fruits and vegetables are all but unknown. Here fish protein is the staff of life. Shark is tough fish and only an aging process makes it edible. Local doctors prescribe it for patients suffering from stomach disorders. Whale steaks are exported to gourmet restaurants and stores throughout this country.

Be happy with such popular menu fish as flounder, mackerel, halibut, perch, trout, bluefish, swordfish. Boiled, baked or fried, they are the epitome of savory dining and add health to you with every morsel. Cold, the next day they make a fine lunch or snack. Shellfish are the gourmet's delight. Rich in minerals and vitamins, and practically all protein, lobsters, crabmeat, clams, and oysters are the crowning eating glory of the fish proteins. Perhaps not priced so reasonably as their underwater cousins with fins, they are a delicious treat at any price.

The Importance of Meat Protein

One of the lowest-priced proteins is chicken. Whether barbecued, roasted, baked, fried or broiled, chicken is an American favorite. Just be careful to avoid those bread crumbs or batters, and the joys of poultry are yours forever.

Some diets forbid meat. Can you imagine having to give up meat altogether? You give up no meat on this diet! *You eat all you want—* steaks, chops, cutlets (no bread crumbs), roasts. You name it. They are all proteins, and all deliciously yours for healthful eating.

The Obesity Builder Doesn't Deal with Proteins

Protein is the only legitimate "miracle" weight-reducer I know. Why anybody would want to spend their money on pills, shots, appetite depressants, and other sometimes dangerous diet drugs to lose weight is beyond my comprehension. Women take green pills to boost their metabolism, red pills to dehydrate themselves, and blue pills to depress themselves. They flood their bodies with these drugs, damaging their organs and their vitality. Little wonder that as soon as they get off the drugs, they gain back all the weight they lost as nature fights to restore depleted organs and wasted tissues. Then the girls are ready for another round. And so goes the obesity mill— grinding out frustrations.

I know women who have had to wait months for appointments with reducing specialists. When they got there, they received a two-minute physical, a taped lecture, and then the boxes of pills. The American Medical Association has been quoted as warning that some patients are being needlessly drugged with possible danger to their health.

Case History of a Model Hurt by Diet Pills

I was surprised to see Miss B. B. She had an 11 A.M. appointment and arrived exactly on time looking like the front cover of a fashion magazine. I guessed her weight at about 115 pounds, and her height at 5′ 5″.

"Don't tell me that you want to lose weight." She told me her problem. She was a model. Her weight was just right, but to keep it that way she was taking so many diet pills that she was quite ill.

I had heard that story many times before. Taking diet pills does not mean that the dieter is eating properly; it just meant that she is not very hungry.

Miss B. B. had developed a habit of having black coffee for breakfast and black coffee for lunch, and she picked at her dinner.

Actually she was somewhat underweight and apart from that had developed some other problems: dizziness, nausea, and pains in her legs—a condition often seen in dieters who lose too much potassium in the process of reducing weight. I sent her to my internist for a check-up. He prescribed high-potency vitamins and minerals. I had to wean her off the diet pills without too much cooperation on her part, as she feared a sudden return of weight. In fact, she did add ten pounds by the time she quit the pills, but lost six of those pounds quickly once her diet was regulated.

She now happily is four pounds more than her original weight and enjoys good health and a calm disposition, and a much better attitude in handling her day-to-day activities.

Dangers of Reducing Exercise Gadgets

Equally futile, albeit not so dangerous as the pills, are the instant reducer exercisers, spot-reducing machines, vibrators and other so-called slenderizing apparatus that offer no permanent weight loss, but only further discourage the already depressed overweight person. Certainly their money goes faster than their excess poundage.

As you read this, women are entering plush reducing salons. They don tights and gym outfits to walk treadmills, chin on bars, pedal machines, roll their bellies and vibrate their hips. From the United States to Japan, Canada to Argentina, women are "getting taken." The gadgets fail dismally. Measurements may change, but the scale proves that the women are just firmer and more fully packed.

I remember hearing of a group of housewives in suburban Boston who formed a neighborhood calisthenics class in the hopes of working off some poundage. Grimly they put each other through the paces, hoping as the weeks passed to acquire figures like movie stars. If they wanted figures like Olympic stars, they would probably still be at it. But the project died for lack of results, and even their newly acquired firmness of flesh soon gave way to their original flabbiness. *They simply ate their flabbiness back fast.*

Even the surgeon's knife has been attempted. Successful plastic surgery has enhanced beauty; why not use it to cut away excess fat? I leave the answer to you.

There are many reasons why women flesh out their big frames or cushion their small ones. Perhaps they gave up smoking and now put food in their mouth instead; or perhaps they never returned to their normal weight after having that second baby; or perhaps it's boredom, or insecurity, or anxiety. But there is only one way to get back to their right weight. *That way is not pounding or perspiring or "pilling." It is not going on starvation diets of carbohydrate-heavy melba toast, cottage cheese and carrot sticks. It is not eating less; it is eating right.*

The obesity mill is a billion-dollar tragedy. Its 50 million victims are bilked out of their money, robbed of their health and tortured in mind and body.

And the answer is so simple and so near. The protein. When I tell women this, I can see them squirm. It is hard to accept the fact that effective dieting can be that easy after one has been through years of its tortuous ups and downs. "But, Mr. Petrie, a doctor gave me those pills. He also gave me printed instructions as to how and when to take each color. How can a licensed physician give you something that is harmful?" My dear lady, the American Medical Association would like the answer to that one, too. Maybe someday somebody will do something about it, but meanwhile as long as there are women who are willing to spend $10 a visit to receive these pills, there will be obesity mills run by doctors who don't mind taking chances with life—the patient's.

What Your Doctor Will Tell You

The family doctor should be consulted before you change your way of eating. Trust him. He agrees with me about these obesity specialists and the harm they can do. He would like you to be able to lose weight because he knows your health will improve. And he will most likely be the first to agree that you should cut out sweets and starches.

How To Make the Easy Transition to the Protein Diet

The high-protein road is an easy one to take and also an easy one to get on. No changes are necessary in your schedule of meals and snacks. I don't care if you eat eight meals a day. Keep it up. But keep the carbohydrate intake down.

If you were sitting in my office for the first time right now, here is what I would tell you to do. Keep on eating exactly the way you would normally eat for the next three days. *But keep a record in writing of everything that you consume.* The time of the meal, the food or beverage, the amount consumed, is important information for you.

This is known as "inventorizing" your eating habits. It provides a visual record of your food consumption. It is a far more accurate way, then relying on memory. It is easy to forget that cookie, that piece of chewing gum, the "coke," or the second portion of cousin Grace's apple pie, that late snack.

This inventory will help to ease you into the high-protein, slimming way of life easily, so easily you won't even notice it.

Before you start the next chapter, inventory at least 24 hours of your eating and drinking. Make the record in column form—left hand column for time, next column for type of food or drink, third column for amount consumed. Leave room for three more columns. I'll tell you what they are for when I see you next.

Review of Chapter Highlights

Identify which of the foods you like are high in protein, low in carbohydrates. Inventory your eating for the next day or two preparatory to making just a few substitutes. High-carbohydrate foods to be avoided are the sweets and starches: potatoes, breads spaghetti, cake, candy, pie. High-protein foods to be enjoyed are meats, eggs, poultry, fish, and cheese.

3

How To Begin the Lazy Lady's Easy Diet
for Permanent Weight Loss

A number of women have told me how they have traveled to a health farm or diet spa to lose weight. They lost as much as 12 pounds in two weeks, only to gain it all back despite a continuing diet soon after they returned home.

The Secret of Losing Pounds Permanently

One formerly vivacious blonde confessed to me that her weight problem was ruining her life. Her doctor insisted that she lose weight. Several trips to a diet farm had provided a sharp weight loss but it was only fleeting success. "You are my last hope; help me," she implored.

I began my first consultation with her with misgivings. Here was a woman who was expecting something dramatic from me, and I did not have even a rainbow-colored pill to offer her. "Forget trips, steam, pounding, pills and all the rest of the show," I said. "Don't expect bells to ring or lights to flash. I'm going to help you. You are going to lose weight and stay thin. But you won't know it's happening." I asked her to bring in a detailed diary of her eating habits for one week (as I set out for you in the previous chapter). She kept elaborate notes. We made exactly four food substitutions and I sent her on her way.

When she returned for her third visit a week later, she looked disappointed. "Why the downcast look?" I asked.

"I lost only two pounds."

"What's wrong with that?"

"But I lost five or six at the diet farm."

"They were different types of pounds," I replied. "Before, you lost 'T' pounds; now, these are 'P' pounds."

"What's the difference?" she asked, feeding me the very line I was fishing to hear from her.

"One's *temporary*, the other *permanent*." She understood at that instant a basic truth about losing weight: *Do it without effort and you do it for good.* She left me 21 pounds later and we both knew she'd never have to be back.

What does this mean to you? It means that the smaller the transition between how you eat now and how you will eat on your easy diet to health and beauty, the more successful you will be.

That is why I asked you to prepare an inventory or diary of your eating habits. I want you to continue those habits with the fewest possible changes. Let's take a look at your record and I'll show you what I mean.

How To Banish Carbohydrate Culprits

By now you should have prepared a chronological schedule of what you ate during a 24-hour period, from the time you rose in the morning to the time you retired at night. If you got out of bed for a snack at 3 A.M. (I knew a woman who kept food by her bed and ate on and off all night) be sure it is recorded on your list. If you thought a hard candy did not count, think again. And put it down. A whiskey sour? On the list it should be.

Now let us see what you have. For purposes of discussion I have reproduced below an actual eating inventory turned in by one of my clients.

Can you tell me anything about this woman? Well, she's a typical business girl who grabs her breakfast on the run. Takes advantage of coffee break time at the office. Eats at a nearby lunch counter. Likes an occasional sweet "Lifesaver" type of candy. Enjoys two cocktails before dinner. Drinks seven—count them—cups of coffee a day. Raids the refrigerator before retiring.

Your inventory is, of course, entirely different. You are a different person. Your time schedule is different. You eat at different places. You cook or order different foods. Maybe you have a cocktail or maybe you have a coke.

7:35 AM	Small orange juice
	1 cup coffee, cream, sugar
10:10 AM	1 prune danish
	1 cup coffee, cream, sugar
	1 Wintergreen Lifesaver
12:20 PM	Cheeseburger
	Apple pie
	2 cups coffee, cream, sugar
	1 mint
	1 Wintergreen Lifesaver
3:40 PM	1 Wintergreen Lifesaver
6:30 PM	2 Whiskey sours
	Sliced London broil
	Home fries
	Peas
	1 portion chocolate cake
	2 cups coffee, cream, sugar
10:50 PM	1 portion chocolate cake
	1 cup coffee, cream, sugar

My interest is in you, not in this career woman we have picked as an example. She has already lost her unwanted weight. You are on the threshold of losing yours. But if you see how we examined her record and what we did about it, you can use the same method with yours.

Did I say: Cut this out, you are eating too much; and then hand her a carbon copy of a standard diet?

I certainly did not. I examined her record with an eye to keeping as much unchanged as was carbohydrate-ly possible. I wanted to make a minimum of changes, yet I had to get her carbohydrate intake below 15 percent (see Chapter 2).

First thing that struck me was the sugar in those seven cups of coffee. What a carbohydrate intake! It had to go! Seven teaspoons of sugar a day are enough carbohydrate hooks for the body to hang fat all the way around its girth and in ever-increasing layers. She turned her nose up when I suggested an artificial sweetener. "Tried them, gives the coffee a different taste." I told her about several persons who had successfully made the transition to sugarless coffee by using lemon for a week. After they stopped squeezing lemon into it, it "tasted sweet" without sugar. No, that sounded too far out to her

Well, then try this and see how it works—use extra sweet cream in every cup. This will serve to sweeten it up without sugar. She agreed to try this. It worked. Then later she cut back on the cream on her own volition, and she made a considerable net carbohydrate saving that way.

How To Handle Coffee-Break Pastries

Next red carbohydrate flag flying on her list was the danish at coffee break. She had this coffee break at her desk. A mobile catering firm arrived with a selection of pastries. Noticing it was prune danish this time, I asked if she ever chose a cheese danish. It was one of her favorites. I prevailed upon her to be her own caterer and bring a few slices of a different cheese every day. It sounded like fun, and she agreed.

How To Eat a Cheeseburger

The cheeseburger came next. Order a double one *without the bread,* I suggested. No argument. And I had her softened up for the next one: Jello, melon, or a raw apple instead of the apple pie. She hesitated. Remember how filling those double cheeseburgers will be. The point was won.

There was still dinner ahead of us. Whiskey sours gave way readily to whiskey on the rocks; the home fries and peas gave way to two vegetables like string beans and broccoli (with Hollandaise sauce). The chocolate cake bowed to custard or any of the gelatin-based desserts now packaged. For the midnight snack, left over London broil would be a premeditated and joyful circumstance.

Menus Compared

Now let's put this new day's menu alongside her old and see how it compares:

	Old Menu	New Menu
7:35 AM	Small orange juice 1 cup coffee, cream, sugar	Small orange juice 1 cup coffee, extra cream
10:10 AM	1 prune danish 1 cup coffee, cream, sugar 1 Wintergreen Lifesaver	Open grilled cheese-sandwich 1 cup coffee, extra cream 1 Wintergreen Lifesaver

12:20 PM	Single cheeseburger on roll	Double cheeseburger, no roll
	Apple pie	Raw apple, two plums
	2 cups coffee, cream, sugar	2 cups coffee, extra cream
	1 Wintergreen Lifesaver	1 Wintergreen Lifesaver
	1 Mint	1 Mint
3:40 PM	1 Wintergreen Lifesaver	1 Wintergreen Lifesaver
6:30 PM	2 Whiskey sours	2 Whiskeys, on rocks
	Sliced London broil	Sliced London broil
	Home fries	Broccoli, Hollandaise
	Peas	String beans
	1 portion chocolate cake	Custard
	2 cups coffee, cream, sugar	2 cups coffee, extra cream
10:50 PM	1 portion chocolate cake	Sliced London broil, cold
	1 cup coffee, cream, sugar	1 cup coffee, extra cream

Not too radically different, is it? Yet the new menu cuts her carbohydrates down to a fraction of what they were. She was eating a total calorie count of 3,570. Her total calorie count is now only 2,182. And look at what has happened to carbohydrate calories. They were 1,389 before. They are 310 now. They were 36 percent of her diet before. They are only 14 percent of her diet now.

This was all the difference between gaining steadily and losing steadily for her. She leveled out seven months later at a slim 48 pounds less.

Put Precious Proteins in Their Right Place in Your Diet

Now we are ready to look at your record. Go about it the same way as I did just before. *Make as few changes as possible,* and attack the highest carbohydrate items first. In the previous case it was the pastry, pie, sugar. What is it in your case? What flour, sugar and other starch are you ready to throw out of your diet.

Sweets and desserts are prime suspects. So are bread, potatoes, soda pop. You don't have to guess. You can figure the calorie value and the carbohydrate value of every food on your list by using the table at the back of this book. List the calorie value and carbohydrate value of each item. Total them up. Put low carbohydrate substitutions and new values in the three columns you left open to the right. Check your new totals. Figure your new percentages. How do they look?

Remember, this is just something you have to do now. You do not count calories forever. But you have to know how to tell the difference between carbohydrate culprits, and precious proteins that help lose unwanted weight. It is easy to tell the difference between a frankfurter and the roll. The precious protein frank stays, the carbohydrate roll is out; don't eat it. (Make it two franks, if you will, but leave the rolls for someone else.) But can you tell whether turnips are a high carbohydrate vegetable, or low? How about spinach, squash, lima beans?

There are low carbohydrate fruits, and high carbohydrate fruits. There are some desserts—for example, zabaglione—that sound rich but are really low in carbohydrates. Knowing their ingredients, you can compute whether they are friend or enemy. The problem of which juices and which beverages are right for you can also be quickly solved.

Tables provide you with an easy reference to decide the substitutions you must make. Work toward the lowest possible carbohydrate values and the highest possible taste value for you. Lowest possible carbohydrate value means taking the weight off. Highest positive taste value means keeping it off.

A Case History of Phenomenal Weight Loss

Sometimes this weight loss is phenomenal. One woman lost 16 pounds the first week. I could not believe my own results, but there she stood on the scale in front of me—all remaining 289 pounds! I must tell you something about this case. Better yet, I'll let her tell you about herself:

"I had made a post-operative gain of 125 pounds in a year's time!

"My ever-increasing girth was actually a lifelong problem, but this tremendous, rapid rise had to be stopped.

"My doctor tried medicines, placebos, etc., but 'no go.' I'd lose one pound and then gain two more. He felt his last resort would be a prolonged hospital stay. I didn't relish the idea even though I needed something drastic. I stopped going to him and kept steadily gaining pounds.

"By this time I'd reached a total of 305 pounds! Since I'm only four feet and seven inches tall, I presented a truly grotesque appearance.

"It was an effort to walk across the street—stairs were impossible. I would sweep the floor sitting on a chair because of the constant agonizing back pain I had.

"Shopping for something to wear became a nightmare. I had to buy the garment because it went on—not because I liked it. There was a stretch of time when it seemed that only blue things were made to fit me.

"By now, other physical conditions were being affected too. Mentally, I was at a low point.

"After Mr. Petrie and I spoke for awhile, he explained how he hoped to help. He had had tremendous success but it was imperative that you work with him.

"Well, the first week I lost 16 pounds!"

The loss did not continue at 16 pounds a week, but it continued favorably downward. *Because she chose her own high-protein foods, she enjoyed her new diet as she lost weight.* And we both knew that she was losing weight permanently. I have enjoyed helping many grossly overweight women and have seen many dramatic transformations, as for example the "before" and "after" photos of Model A.

How To Count the Carbohydrates in a Meal

The calorie table at the back of the book gives you an instant carbohydrate count on the most common foods, all by average portion. You can total the carbohydrate foods in any day's menu, item by item. You can also total the full calorie count, item by item. Then you can divide the latter into the former for a percentage figure to see if you are under your 15 percent carbohydrate allowance, as discussed in Chapter 2.

How To Figure a Reducing Breakfast

Take a simple breakfast as an example: a large glass of orange juice, English muffin and coffee. The following values are taken from the table:

	CARBOHYDRATE CALORIES	TOTAL CALORIES
Orange juice, 1 cup (8 oz.)	80	80
English muffin, large	184	280
Butter, 1 tablespoon	——	101
Coffee, 1 cup	——	——
Cream, 1 tablespoon	2	29
	266	490

This is a 490-calorie breakfast with a total of 266 of those calories being carbohydrates. Divide 490 into 266 and you get .54 or 54 percent.

Now this is a breakfast you will want to do something about. It is a fattening breakfast. It has three or four times as much carbohydrate calories as it should have.

What do you do about it? Do you skip breakfast altogether? Starve yourself for the first few hours of the day? This is the answer that many women arrive at. *But it is the wrong answer, as their continuing weight problem bears witness to.*

The right answer is to eat a nourishing breakfast but one that is low in fattening carbohydrates. The right answer for you is to make as few changes as possible in the breakfast you enjoy, substituting even more enjoyable dishes for the carbohydrate dishes you abandon.

If the foregoing breakfast was your favorite breakfast, you would try to limit substitutions to one or two if possible to transform it into a weight-loss breakfast. Obviously, the English muffin is the culprit. One substitution will do the trick. Put a protein food in its place and your carbohydrate calories will be contained mostly in the large eight-ounce glass of orange juice.

Can I talk you into an order of bacon and eggs? How about a rasher of Canadian bacon? It all takes too much time in the morning, you say. And it also dirties a frying pan. Well, how about putting those delicious eggs up before you put the water on to boil. And did you know that the new coated cookwear cleans with a good rinse?

A Secretary's Experience with a Hot Breakfast

A twenty-eight-year-old secretary to a television executive told me she had agreed to try a hot breakfast just to please me, but wound up pleasing herself. "The first day I set the alarm clock 15 minutes early to play safe," she said, "but then I found I was ready to leave the apartment 15 minutes before time." She told me how the aroma of frying bacon and the crackling of eggs in the pan has now become "an important part of waking up." Looking back at the English muffin, she wondered how it could have been satisfying to her.

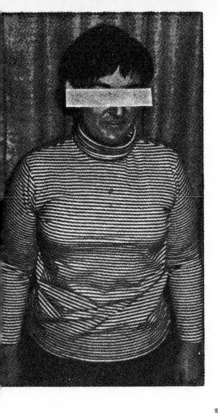

Model A, After

Model A, Before

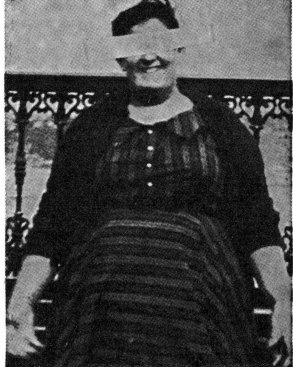

How To Liven Your Breakfast Planning for Weight Loss

There are many delicious breakfast meats. Sausages come pre-cooked and need only to be browned. Luncheon meat like Spam is a quickie breakfast, too. Hash, ham steak, take a few minutes more.

Add variety to your breakfast fare. Switch to several of the many high-protein meats. Or consider the smoked, salted or creamed fish that the British are so fond of for breakfast. Even cheese is on their breakfast menus.

They all add up to zero carbohydrates. In some there is a trace of carbohydrates, but not enough to affect totals or percentages. Consider them as perfect substitutes for the carbohydrated foods you want to banish once and for all.

An eight-ounce glass of orange juice is rather large and filling. With a lusty breakfast of bacon and eggs you will probably be satisfied with a smaller glass of juice, say a four- or six-ounce glass. Orange juice is an excellent food for beauty and health. A carbohydrate calorie of orange juice is worth its weight in vitamins and minerals.

Reduce rather than replace some items that are being consumed in over-normal portions, especially fruits and vegetables that are high in nutrients. Guidance in recognizing these youth-full foods is in the chapters ahead. Save your carbohydrate quotas for these foods. Be unrelenting with foods that are sweet and starchy just for the sake of being sweet and starchy.

This sample breakfast has been easy to figure and easy to transform. It has taken only one basic substitution to make it a healthful, slimming way of starting the day. And most important, the substitution has meant more delicious food to eat, not less.

Compute the carbohydrate calories and total calories of every item of intake on your inventory or diary you prepared at the start of this chapter. Add your totals. Compute your percentages. Then make telling substitutions.

A Search for Camouflaged Carbohydrates Pays Off

I remember the time when a thirty-five-year-old school teacher arrived for her appointment after one week of dining on her new protein fare. She had made her own substitutions, going along the lines I prescribed. Yet the needle on the scale had not budged.

We reviewed the previous twenty-four eating hours together. She had hash for breakfast. Lunch had consisted of mushroom soup, a Caesar salad. Dinner included fried chicken. These were minimum carbohydrate foods—corned beef hash, mushrooms, cheese-dressed salad, chicken. She had other side dishes of fruits and vegetables which she had computed at about the 15 percent level. Her figures were right, but there just had to be some serious omissions. So I dug for them with a few culinary questions as follows: (a) Was the hash mostly potatoes? (b) Was the mushroom soup thickened with flour? (c) Did the Caesar salad have a liberal sprinkling of croutons? (d) Was the chicken dropped in a batter before frying? The answers were yes, yes, yes, and yes; and the four yes's added up to an esti- mated 250 carbohydrate calories. All excess hooks to hang un- wanted pounds on.

Now these excess carbohydrates can have a disastrous effect on the whole program. Eat-all-you-want goes out the window if you supply your body with carbohydrate hooks to store surpluses. Where would the eat-all-you-want restaurants be if they supplied containers to take out what you could not consume? Bankrupt. And that is what extra carbohydrate calories do to a good figure. They bankrupt it!

Did you know that veal cutlets were just as delicious *without the breading?* And cream cheese cake just as velvety smooth *without the graham cracker crust?* The path to permanent weight loss and a slender figure is along the gourmet trail of fun eating only *if you sidestep carbohydrates.*

Researchers at a New York university recently found that the carbohydrate and insulin abnormalities of obese persons can begin in childhood. On the basis of preliminary experimental work with animals, they found indications that excess eating during infancy establishes adipose (fat) cells which later are able to store fat. When the individual matures, all it takes is some sweet and starch to start the pound count ascending by filling these cells.

Carbohydrate Calories over 300 Are Too Many for One Day

That is one of the reasons why some people have to watch carbo- hydrates less carefully than others. They were thin babies. Obvi- ously you are not one of those people or you probably would not have a weight problem. Your war, though, is not against food, or good food and adequate amounts of it. *Your war is against carbo-hydrates.* You must root out every excess carbohydrate calorie to enjoy eating while you get slim. And, therefore, to stay slim. *Reminder: excess carbohydrates are every blessed carbohydrate calorie over 300.* Call 250 to 300 per day a minimum requirement. Call every other one, calorie non gratis, and don't welcome any more into your body, and you'll be glad you did!

Recipes which use sweet wines, bread crumbs, flour, sugar, need to be altered to eliminate these carbohydrate-heavy ingredients or at least to drastically curtail them.

You don't have to make any great sacrifices to change our school teacher's four yes's into four no's. Corned beef hash is great without potatoes—or make hash from leftover ground steak with a fraction of a potato. Mushroom soup tastes even more delicious when thickened with cream instead of flour. Caesar salad is just as interesting without croutons added. Chicken fried "nude" in the fat is every bit as good as when encrusted in batter, and will be better for you.

How To Eat Like a Gourmet and Lose Unwanted Pounds

To make gourmet dieting an even easier reality for you, I have revised a number of exotic recipes to eliminate or minimize carbo-hydrate content without affecting their enjoyment value. Appendix I contains about 100 low-carbohydrate recipes. Included are soups, salads, omelettes, entrees, desserts—all you need to put zest into your dining as you eat your weight away.

Note that each of the recipes is evaluated for carbohydrate and total calories per portion. Note also that the carbohydrate calories never exceed 15 percent. Do the same with your own favorite recipes. Take out carbohydrates, put in flavorings, sauces, spices. Then add up the carbohydrate calories and total calories. If they pass the 15 percent test, put them in the front of your file.

To help in menu planning, a list of food reminders for every meal is given in Table 2. You can pick one item from each list and form an almost endless variety of daily menus. They all make healthful, slenderizing meals. Use your own ingenuity to add to each list for breakfast, lunch or dinner. Go short on carbohydrates, long on pleasure of eating—and melt the pounds away through the Easy Diet.

BUILD YOUR MENUS FROM THIS
STARTING LIST

Breakfast	Lunch	Dinner
Grapefruit	Consommé	Chopped liver
Orange juice	Tomato soup	Shrimp cocktail
Tomato juice	Cream of mushroom	Baked clams
Prune juice	Lobster bisque	Ham prosciutto
Blackberry juice		
Sauerkraut juice	Chicken salad	Oysters
	Egg salad	Fowl (any type)
Eggs any style	Shrimp salad	roasted, baked,
Bacon	Tuna fish salad	broiled
Canadian bacon	Ham salad	Roast beef
Ham	Hamburger steak	Roast lamb
Scrapple	Frankfurters	Roast pork (any cut)
Sausage	Omelettes any style	Broiled steak (any
Luncheon meat		cut)
	Tangerine	Broiled fish (any type)
Coffee	Rhubarb	
Tea	Cheese	Asparagus
	Jello	Cabbage
		Celery
	Coffee	Mushrooms
	Tea	Turnip greens
		Spinach
		String beans
		Melon
		Strawberries, whipped
		cream
		Custard
		Zabaglione
		Coffee
		Tea

Table 2

Review of Chapter Highlights

Substitute high-protein foods for the high-carbohydrate foods on your dietary diary. Count carbohydrate calories and keep them around 15 percent of total calories. Make as few changes as possible by cutting only the worst offending foods. The more you wring out excess carbohydrates, the more you can eat and the faster you will lose weight.

4

Delicious Foods That Bring You Better
Health and a Beautiful Figure

Happiness for a lot of women is trying on a size-14 dress and finding it is a mite too big. Happiness is also passing up a piece of cake because you really don't want or need it. Happiness is enjoying a steak dinner and knowing it won't make a permanent bulge on your body. Happiness is being able to touch your toes and not bend your knees. Happiness is having men turn to look at you.

The way to happiness has been opened to you. It is a way that thousands of women have successfully taken. It is a fun way—with tempered judgment, rather than grinding discipline. It is a way to permanent happy results—via habit instead of diet.

Eating more, instead of less, and losing weight in the process has one other tremendous advantage over starvation and deprivation in a "diet." You can eat *more* of the beauty and health foods instead of less of them.

Of course, no matter how you lose weight, your health will improve. "I have lost 11 pounds in two months," one woman writes. "I have not dieted rigidly or skipped meals, but I eat more high-protein foods. I feel immensely better; it's like I lost many more pounds, and years off my age."

How To Get Hooked on Diets and Reducing Workouts

The will to diet is, for most people, wishful shrinking. They put it off and put it off. Finally they take the distasteful plunge. For days,

41

maybe weeks, they torture themselves and "take it out" on their family and friends. But the *body beautiful* they seek remains the *body bountiful.*

The next stop is the steam room, where they actually pay good money to a masseur or masseuse to be pummeled, slammed and mauled.

Or they will join other larded ladies in group-therapy types of you-watch-my-weight-and-I'll-watch-your-weight sessions.

Maybe something will happen. Maybe they will lose meaningful poundage. But we all know the end of the story. *There are more diets in their future, more pummeling and more therapy* without a foreseeable end.

The ups and downs of weight gain and weight loss are not health-ful. The end result of weight loss is healthful, but the losing process —especially if rapid—is a risky matter and anybody will tell you that to do so without being under a doctor's supervision is asking for trouble. Think of the strain the body suffers when subjected to crash diet after crash diet separated by carbohydrate-rich periods of weight gain.

How To Get Un-Hooked on Diets and Reducing Nostrums

To lose weight gradually and permanently is triple insurance. It avoids radical changes in diet that can deprive the body of essential nutrients. It avoids the constant instability of cycles of weight loss and weight gain that can rob the body of youth and vitality. It avoids extended periods of overweight in between diets that rob years from life expectancy.

Let us go one step further. *Let us eat right as we eat well to lose weight.* This chapter will help you make the substitutions of high-protein for high-carbohydrate foods that you have now begun in such a way that the most valuable foods for bodily health are in-cluded. I promise that these foods will not be of the cottage cheese and carrot stick variety. They will be as delicious as the other gourmet foods already slated to be a permanent way of life. Read on and see.

The "Stuff" of Life

There was a time when wheat was one of the sole foods on which men could rely during many months of the year. Bread became known as the "staff of life."

Now, this term came along many centuries before man knew about nutrition. Yet, by some strange accuracy, the proper designation of "staff" was chosen, meaning something to lean on. It would have been inaccurate to call bread the "stuff" of life, for carbohydrate is a staff on which man can lean temporarily for energy and survival.

We now know that of all the three ingredients in natural food—carbohydrate, fat, and protein—*only protein is indispensable.* Protein is the only one of the three foods that has nitrogen in it. All living material is composed of protein, with nitrogen bound into its organic molecules. *So it is really protein that deserves to be called the "stuff" of life.*

Protein Is Essential to Life

The ability of the body to synthesize what it needs from the food we eat is uncanny. A mixed diet of various carbohydrate and protein foods will give the body all it needs to maintain healthy tissue, flesh, bone, blood and organs. The fat will not be missed. A mixed diet of fat and protein foods will do likewise. The carbohydrate will not be missed. But a mixed diet of carbohydrates and fats will not sustain the body. The proteins will be vitally missed.

I do not advocate trying to do without carbohydrates entirely. It would be almost impossible, but if you could, you might disturb the body's metabolic process. People who have dropped their carbohydrate intake to less than 200 carbohydrate calories have shown a tendency to develop acetones, a symptom often found in diabetics.

I do advocate limiting carbohydrates to 15 percent of your calorie intake, and substituting the "stuff" of life in their place—protein.

Besides building flesh and blood, proteins enable the body to build cells known as phagocytes or antibodies. They destroy bacteria and viruses. They are the most essential key to bodily resistance to disease. It is a matter of record that increasing the protein content of a diet can cause the body to produce as much as a hundred times more antibodies.

Your Internal 30-Foot Conveyor Belt and How To Make It Work for Your Health

The body has a 30-foot conveyor belt to process the food that you feed it, your gastrointestinal tract. An involved chemical conversion takes place, starting with the saliva at the intake end of the system, your mouth, and continuing with the hydrochloric acid and pepsin in the stomach. Carbohydrates advance along the conveyor belt fastest. Proteins are slower, while fats are slower still.

As the material leaves the stomach and enters the small intestine, the alkaline secretions of the liver and pancreas go to work. Bile and pancreatic juice neutralize the acid and then enzymes break the food down further, and many now begin to release their nutrients. Cellulose and fats still resist, but they too will soon be conquered.

It takes the conveyor belt four to eight hours more to move the food through the small intestine, where it is churned by waves of movement called peristalsis and swished through millions of tiny fingers that both stir and transfer nutrients into the lymph and blood systems.

Finally, a 10- to 12-hour trip through the large intestine subjects what is left of the food to attack by large colonies of bacteria. This produces the final decay and the material exits through the colon.

Thus are carbohydrates and fats converted into simple energy sources and proteins into the basic building material of the body, called amino acids.

I would like to come back a moment to those millions of fingers in the small intestine. They are nearly microscopic and are called villi. They have hungry mouths seeking minerals, vitamins and basic elements required by the body. These materials are the special building blocks of the body, as compared to the basic building blocks—the protein-derived amino acids.

If the food does not contain these special building blocks, the million little fingers with mouths in them go hungry—or you might say empty-handed. The body begins to lack essential nutrients. Nails break, flesh sags, skin wilts, hair dulls. Vital organs lose their vitality. The body's resistance to disease lowers.

Is there room for sufficient foods with high nutrition value on a starvation diet? The answer is no. That is why it is called a starvation diet. Will enough nutritious foods fit on the usual 1,000-calorie crash program diet? The answer is still no. Most people on these crash programs must take concentrated vitamin and mineral supplements to prevent bodily deterioration. Will enough nutritious foods fit on a 15 percent carbohydrate diet? The answer is yes. And since you can eat more total calories on a low carbohydrate diet and still lose weight, you can eat more of those total nutrients that the body continuously needs.

Key Nutrients Are in Vegetables

This is not a book on nutrition. There are plenty of expert nutritionists who have written on the subject. I have researched much of what has been done in this field and continue to keep an eye on latest findings.

So I am able to highlight for you what I find to be the soundest nutritional information obtainable. I use the word "obtainable," because I do not feel man knows enough today about the food he eats and the needs of his body. Nor do I feel he is making good progress in this space age about such down-to-earth matters.

A study of digestion was made by a young Army surgeon, Dr. William Beaumont, in 1822 and is still considered a masterpiece today. Dr. Beaumont used as his subject a fur trapper whose stomach wall had been shot away. He was able to perform experiments in gastric digestion, making observations through the stomach wall.

Folk medicine is replete with natural cures that were once looked on as superstition by the medical profession and are now known to be valid uses of sources of therapeutic chemicals. In fact, one might call the preoccupation of today's botanists and scientists with old books or curative herbs a remarkable turnabout. In the book *Nature's Medicines*,[1] Richard Lucas traces herbal remedies that man has used since the dawn of recorded history and tells how many have led to today's prescriptions.

Nature grows everything needed by man. Fruits and vegetables are a good start in the direction of good nutrition. They contain the enzymes, vitamins, and minerals that fortify and beautify the body. See the book *Helping Your Health with Enzymes*,[2] by C. Wade for a complete rundown on enzymes.

Take the lowly mushroom. Dr. L. R. Hesler, retired dean emeritus of the University of Tennessee College of Liberal Arts, has worked with mushrooms for thirty years and recently found different chemicals in the mushroom cap from which antibiotics may be developed. Mushrooms are important to the natural life cycle, Dr. Hesler says, because they live on dead and decaying materials. They are high on

---

[1] Richard Lucas, *Nature's Medicines* (West Nyack, N.Y.: Parker Publishing Company, Inc., 1966).
[2] C. Wade, *Helping Your Health with Enzymes* (West Nyack, N.Y.: Parker Publishing Company, Inc.)

my list of recommended vegetables because they taste good, they are good for you, and they are low in carbohydrate calories and in total calories.

Notice I place taste first on the list. I consider it a useless bit of advice to recommend as healthful something that does not taste good. If you don't like it, it has no place on your permanent, slimming diet. Of what value is it to you if I tell you that raw yeast is one of the most healthful of vegetables—richest source of B vitamins and also rich in alkaline elements like potassium and sodium—if you don't like raw yeast, and few people do.

Most vegetables taste good. Lowest in calories, including carbohydrates, are the leafy vegetables—lettuce, Chinese cabbage, spinach, kale, collard, etc. Include in this category the so-called greens like watercress, dandelion greens, endive, chives, mustard greens, parsley.

Also low in total calories and carbohydrates are the bud vegetables like cabbage and brussel sprouts. A stem-and-bud vegetable that is one of the lowest in carbohydrates is asparagus. Most of the stem or tuber vegetables are to be avoided: potatoes, kohlrabi, Jerusalem artichokes. Ditto most of the root vegetables, which are also fairly high in carbohydrates, like beets, sweet potatoes, yams, rutabagas. Not quite so high are their brothers, the carrots, parsnips, turnips and radishes.

Many fruits of plants are called vegetables. Look each one up on the carbohydrate calorie tables or on the menu charts before deciding whether it belongs on your shopping list. They include cucumbers, squash, eggplant, tomatoes, zucchini, lima beans, peppers, okra and string beans.

Grains and cereals are the seeds of plants and we seldom refer to them as vegetables. They are high in carbohydrate calories, especially in refined and prepared forms, as are their more common vegetable confreres such as corn, rice, beans, peas and lentils.

Now let us see what nutrients the body needs and in which of these vegetables we may find them.

How To Find Life-Giving Substances in Food

"Vitamin" is a name given to substances found in natural foods that seem to be essential to the life, or physiological functions, of man and animals. So complex are these substances that even scientists prefer to call them by their alphabetical designations than their chemical names. Vitamin A, B, C, D, E, F, G, K and P are a lot easier to cope with than such names as para-aminobenzoic acid. And where different types have been discovered within a lettered category, it has been a simple matter to drag out numbers to tag them with.

Vitamin A

Without it: Impairment of bone formation; defective teeth and teeth enamel; night blindness; deficiencies in skin, digestive system, respiratory tract, genitourinary system.

With it: Vigorous new cell growth, high resistance to infections, a delay in senility and increase in longevity.

Get it from: Dandelion greens, turnip greens, spinach, collard, kale, mustard greens, broccoli, squash. Also calf's liver.

Vitamin B1 (Thiamine)

Without it: Lack of ability to concentrate, lack of energy, fatigue, irritability, loss of appetite, distension of abdomen, retarded growth, loss of muscular tone, dry hair.

With it: Smooth functioning digestive system, healthy appetite, proper heart rhythm, normal growth and muscular tone.

Get it from: Brewer's yeast, soybean flour, turnip greens, peas, wheat germ, brown rice. Also beef heart and beef kidney.

Vitamin B2

Without it: Visual difficulties, corneal vascularization, digestive disturbances, nervous depression, loss of hair, fingernail changes, dermatitis, diminished vitality, lowered resistance to infection, early aging.

With it: Proper functioning of gastrointestinal tract, longer duration of virility and fertility.

Get it from: Turnip greens, Brewer's yeast, wheat germ, peas. Also beef liver, kidney and heart.

Vitamin B—Niacin

Without it: Pellagra and diseases of the central nervous system.

With it: Normal metabolism, oxidation of carbohydrates, growth.

Get it from: Peanut butter, turnip greens, peas, wheat germ. Also calf's liver, red salmon.

Vitamin C (Ascorbic Acid)

Without it: Soft and bleeding gums, lack of endurance, listlessness, retarded growth, scurvy.

With it: Healthy teeth and gums, prompt healing of mucous tissue, efficient cell respiration and oxidation; stimulated production of bone marrow and cortical hormones.

Get it from: Rose hip marmalade, broccoli, turnip greens, collards, green pepper, mustard greens. Also, citrus fruits and strawberries.

Vitamin D

Without it: Inability to absorb calcium from foods.
With it: Good bone structure, especially in later years.
Get it from: Sunshine. No foods contain significant amounts.

Vitamin E

Without it: Muscular wasting, an increased need for oxygen by the tissues.
With it: Regeneration of the muscles, improved heart condition.
Get it from: Corn oil, wheat germ oil, soy oil, cottonseed oil, kale, corn, spinach, brussel sprouts. Also most meats.

Vitamin F (fatty acids)

Without it: Tendency to arteriosclerosis.
With it: Proper maintenance of blood cholesterol level, body warmth.
Get it from: Wheat germ oil, corn oil, soy oil.

Vitamin K

Without it: Hemorrhaging
With it: Proper coagulation of the blood.
Get it from: Spinach, cabbage, cauliflower, tomato.

Get the Most Good from the Least Food

The sources listed for each of the vitamins are those in which that vitamin is found in the most concentrated quantities. They do not have a monopoly on those vitamins. All fresh vegetables have vitamins; all fresh fruits have vitamins. Freezing does not destroy the vitamins. Canning takes a heavy toll. Cooking, too. The more freshly picked the higher the vitamin content. The closer to peak ripeness or maturity the higher the vitamin content.

I often wonder if I will ever meet someone who has had the opportunity to eat turnip greens every day fresh and raw right out of the garden. That person should be glowing with health.

But also glowing with that fresh and crisp look of vibrance will be all those persons who spike their daily menus with a liberal quota of cool salads, green vegetables and savory fruits.

How much does the body need of these magic alphabetized substances? Two servings a day of greens, such as spinach, mustard, turnip, will provide you with several times the minimum requirements of Vitamin A recommended by nutritionists.

Broiled liver twice a week, or a tablespoon of yeast several times a week in gravies or stews, or a sprinkling of wheat germ over hot cereal, or in place of bread crumbs when cooking, will in themselves provide plenty of Vitamin B in your diet. Those green Vitamin A sources are working for you here, too.

Fresh citrus fruits and leafy vegetables once or twice a day provide a generous allowance of Vitamin C.

Vitamin D will be in the eggs you eat for breakfast and in tuna and salmon, even canned. The other vitamins have a good chance of arriving in the quantities you need in the same foods that carry their alphabetical predecessors.

People who eat in restaurants most of the time, or you girls who have not yet developed a taste for salads and greens, had best supplement their diet with high-quality vitamin tablets and capsules. They will add many youthful years to your life span.

Canning of foods has made great progress and more of the nutrients are retained than a decade ago. But there is still a substantial loss compared to garden-fresh vegetables. The cooking process is the greatest enemy of the vitamin. It is not so much the heat as the water. Vitamins are water soluble and when vegetables are cooked in water the vitamins wind up down the drain with the water residue.

Women are now becoming more and more aware of the watery escape path taken by vitamins. They save these vegetable liquors and use them in soups, gravies and sauces. They also try to use less water when cooking.

Summing up on vitamins: In substituting high-protein foods for high-carbohydrate foods, try to include a daily portion of green leafy vegetables, a daily citrus fruit or its juice, and a weekly portion of liver or other organ meats. A diversified menu, fresh, air, pure water and sunshine will take care of the balance of your health requirements with one exception—the need for minerals.

A Mine for Minerals Is at Your Supermarket

The body requires minerals both for its structure and the proper functioning of that structure. These minerals build bone, teeth, nails, hair and muscle. They help control acidity and alkalinity.

They act as catalysts in promoting vital chemical reactions. They are vital to the conductivity of nerve tissue in message sending. They help maintain water levels so necessary to life processes. They play important roles in drawing other nutrients into the body. They help muscles to exert their strength.

Chief among these minerals are calcium, phosphorus, iron, copper, manganese, iodine, potassium and sodium. Traces of many more minerals are found in the body and undoubtedly play key parts in the body's healthful functioning, but they are absorbed by the body in sufficient quantity from the same foods that supply the chief minerals and vitamins needed.

You cannot walk into a supermarket and buy minerals packaged, priced and ready for the check-out counter. Yet the minerals are there in abundance, waiting to do their work in bringing women radiant health and exuberance. They are in the dairy department, the vegetable bins and the fish and meat departments. Let's check each mineral, noting as we did in the case of vitamins, what they do and where they can be found.

Calcium

What it does: Helps build teeth, bones and nails. Aids in nerve transmission, which in turn promotes sound sleep and feelings of all's well with the world. Assists muscles to function properly, minimizing muscular cramps, including abdominal cramps during menstruation.

Where it can be found: Milk, most cheeses, except cottage, dark molasses, dried dates and figs, green vegetables and tops, seafood, egg yolk, olives.

Phosphorus

What it does: Works like calcium and often in conjunction with it for bones, teeth, muscle, nerves and glands.

Where it can be found: Cheese, most nuts, peas, beans, lentils, saltwater fish, unrefined grains, all meats and poultry.

Iron

What it does: Enables the blood to carry essential oxygen throughout the body, prevents anemia and listlessness, helps remove carbon dioxide from body cells, contributes to quick thinking and mental alertness.

Where it can be found: Liver, fresh meats, green vegetables and avocados, oysters, egg yolk, molasses, bran, apricots, celery, soy-beans, wheat germ.

Copper manganese

What it does: Works hand in glove with iron.
Where it can be found: Basically the same foods as iron, also huckleberries, oatmeal.

Iodine

What it does: Essential to the functioning of the thyroid gland, which supplies stamina and vitality for work and play.
Where it can be found: Ocean fish, shellfish, iodized salt.

Potassium

What it does: Essential to muscle action, including heart function-ing, and bowel evacuation.
Where it can be found: Whole-grain cereals, molasses, green leafy vegetables.

Sodium

What it does: Aids normal digestion of protein, assists absorption of other minerals into blood.
Where it can be found: Usually contained in sufficient amounts in normally salted food, together with chlorine needed by the body for hydrochloric acid used in the stomach digestive process. Should be used more in hot weather to compensate for loss due to perspiration, except as otherwise advised by physician.

Again we find that our high-protein diet provides us with the minerals we need and all we have to remember to include in the daily menu are those green leafy vegetables. Fish, cheese, meat and eggs—all basic foods on our high protein menu—supply necessary amounts of these important–to–you minerals.

Since you can eat more the high-protein way, and still not gain weight, you can maintain an exuberantly high level of youthful health, femininity and charm.

Dieting for Health

You still see a figure of 40 million mentioned as the number of overweight people in the United States. But that was a 1960 esti-mate. Despite the passion to lose weight in recent years, the number of overweight people has now grown to over 75 million. These are the people who are padded enough to be concerned with their

weight as a problem with which they must cope. The major reason
their ranks are growing, besides our carbohydrate way of life, is
that, though many lose weight, they rejoin the ranks of the overweight soon again.

I alone through my writings, radio and television appearances
have probably convinced more than 100,000 of these concerned
people to go protein. The new popularity of this old tried and true
concept is being expanded by other writers and nutritionists. Undoubtedly there are now millions of overweight people who are on
the protein path and are leaving the ranks of the overweight, never
to swell them again.

I was particularly gratified to learn recently that several hospitals
have adopted the low-carbohydrate diet for their patients. Greater
medical acceptance, however, will always be tempered with the
need to treat each person individually, and I agree wholeheartedly
with this. One woman's elixir can be another woman's poison. Just
as carbohydrates or fats can be dangerous to persons with certain
physical problems, proteins can also be dangerous in isolated cases.

But injections and pills are dangerous in more than just isolated
cases. When a woman walks into my office for assistance in losing
weight, I can tell by her appearance if she has been on appetite
depressant, desiccants, pep pills or other medication to lose weight.
They are wan and drawn-looking. Their skin is dull and sallow.
They are nervous, irritable, ill at ease.

Do they look this way on fish, meat, salads, eggs, cheeses and
greens? What a difference! They stand straighter, walk more vigorously and seem to have a new lease on life. They have a healthy skin
tone. They radiate good health.

Take another look at your eating record and the substitutions of
protein food you have made. Are all of the vitamins and minerals
sources on there? If not, make another substitution or two to make
sure you are giving yourself your full share of nature's never-ending
source-spring of youth.

Review of Chapter Highlights

Include your favorite vitamin- and mineral-rich foods on your
shopping lists. Key nutrients are in vegetables, especially the leafy
kinds. For beauty and health, check those foods high in vitamins A,
B, C, D, E, F, G, K, and P; also enjoy foods high in minerals like
calcium, phosphorus, iron, copper manganese, iodine, potassium,
and sodium.

5

How Eating the Right Foods Can Make

You More Beautiful

Let us set down what we have covered in this book so far:

1. We will make as few changes as possible in our old diet so that our new diet will be easier to stay on permanently.
2. Since carbohydrate foods are the most fattening of all foods, we will substitute something else in their place, making fewest changes.
3. Since protein foods are the most essential to the body, and the least fattening, we will use them as the substitutes, down to only 15 percent carbohydrate intake.
4. Protein foods are largely meat, fish, cheese, eggs and poultry.
5. Good health also depends on a diversified diet of vitamins and minerals, chiefly found in citrus fruits, organ meats and fresh greens.

In this chapter, I will show you how the low carbohydrate diet can pay off in woman's most cherished dream—being more beautiful.

Women think they can buy a good figure. They try to attain the 36-24-36 measurement by hook, crook, prop, pad, lace and elastic. They think they can buy a pretty face. They paint, shade, powder, cream, add attachments, and they think they can buy beautiful hair. They dye, tint, wash, spray, and then cover it all with a wig!

Beauty is closer to you than you think. Certainly it is closer than the corner drug store. It is in your own home, and it is more likely to be in the kitchen than in the bathroom, but even more likely to be already within you—waiting to come through.

How To Get the Ideal Female Body Dimensions

Men hate the "girdled look." You can have perfect dimensions, but if they exist through force and pressure of undergarment, a man *knows* it is artificial. If a 37-24-37 dream walks by without a natural jiggle, a man sees not a girl, but a well-plated battle wagon.

The world will never know how many marriages were wrecked, jobs lost, friendships broken, and lives jeopardized by bulging, bad figures. I know that my own files show how a few inches here and there have brought fantastic success endings to stories that were headed for the tragedy pit—ex-stars of stage and screen who made comebacks, frustrated career girls who made it to the top, older women who found a new zest for living, unworkable marriages that turned into love affairs.

Is the classic 36-24-36 figure right for you? The answer is "not necessarily so." No two women are alike, and only nature knows the right dimensions for you. Give nature a chance and you will have those dimensions. They might be 36-24-35 or 35-24-36. You might be naturally a size 10, but then again you might be a size 6 or a size 14 at your natural best.

If you lose weight on pills that dehydrate your body, you are not even giving nature half a chance. Mother Nature must restore your body fluids just as soon as you turn off the dehydrating pressure that was generated by drugs. If you lose weight by mechanical vibrator, she will also work to restore muscle, fat and tissue in the areas where unnatural applicators have worked them off.

But eat wholesome foods, free of fattening carbohydrate excesses, and nature restores your figure to its natural best. She takes the pounds off where they need to come off to restore the real you to your own beautiful form.

Nature's wisdom is beyond comprehension by us. Can you imagine what women would look like if there were certain ways to diet to take pounds off the bust and other ways that would take pounds off the hips or thighs or stomach or buttocks. Women would overdo it here and underdo it there. They would emerge from such diet sprees in distorted shapes just as when they emerge from the corset shop.

There are, fortunately, no such ways to diet. No local or regional reducing is possible through diet. And the opposite is also true. You cannot put weight on where you think you need it to the exclusion of the rest of your anatomy.

Nature has decreed that you are always you. The silhouette that you make, the features that you present, are what define you to everyone else. Every leaf on a tree is different from the next, and each is as beautiful as the next. The real, natural you is a beautiful person. To paraphrase a famous statement: Inside every unattractive, overweight woman is a beautiful, slender one trying to get out.

How We Interfere with Natural Beauty

The body is a work of art. It is capable of the most remarkable feats. The ballet dancer, the acrobat, the athlete exploits these miraculous attributes of the physical organism we call our body. The majority of the rest of us appear to do everything we can to "hush up" the body. We let it sit most of the time. We seldom extend any of its muscles or exercise its skills. We don't even make reasonable efforts to hold it erect.

If anybody were to ask me what, next to carbohydrates, contributed most to unattractiveness, I would without hesitation reply— *posture*.

I mean this word "posture" in two different ways. I mean it in the usual way, where bad posture is the slumping, tummy out, shoulders drooped stance; and good posture is the gracefully straight, erect, all's-right-with-the-world stance.

I also mean the word posture to indicate an attitude toward life. If we have an all's-wrong-with-the-world feeling, we are not going to portray anything different in the way we look. We will stand stooped as if the burdens of the world were on our shoulders and we will have a down-in-the-mouth expression on our face.

The two meanings of the word posture are therefore quite related and we cannot very well speak of standing posture and ignore the philosophical posture. This philosophical posture is one of the greatest obstacles that we place in nature's path to beauty.

It is a simple matter to substitute proteins for carbohydrates, but how does one go about substituting a positive posture for a negative one? Any one of my 1,000 women can tell you. It is one of the first things we do once the carbohydrate culprits are handcuffed and led away. It has not much to do with food, but unless you correct the bad food habits, the good posture will be next to impossible.

How a Positive Beauty Posture Can Be Obtained

Poor nutrition walks hand in hand with poor posture. Indeed, one seems to accelerate the other. Lack of proteins and minerals weak ens the muscles and tissues and leads to poor posture. This in turn creates a depressed feeling and a depressed look. Poor posture hinders circulation, thus further depriving the body of the nutrition it needs.

Your posture is already improved if you have made "protein for carbohydrate" switches on your menu, and if you have included the vitamin and mineral foods, too. You know you are losing weight. You know you are on the road to greater beauty and you are proud and erect.

How Posture Guided a Mother to Weight Reduction

One thirty-eight-year-old mother of three weighed in at 174 pounds, and stood 5 feet 3 in her stocking feet. She had a pretty face, but it looked like it was painted on a blimp. Two weeks later she had lost eight pounds and was convinced that she was now on her way to her former beauty. She walked with a more buoyant step, held her head high and her shoulders back. When I called her attention to this, she replied, "I have a new outlook on life. I realize that my fat was making an old woman of me before my time. Now I realize I am still young, with my life still ahead of me." Three months later she had lost 40 pounds, some nine inches from her abdomen and seven inches from her hips. She had real reason then to walk lightly, head up, but her anticipation helped to assure the successful attainment of her goal.

An overweight woman loses respect for herself. She realizes she is not attractive. She begins to let herself go in many ways. She burns with envy at her svelte counterparts. She despises her own lack of willpower and her repeated failures.

How Overweight Helps Undermine Morale and Beauty

One such "hefty" wrote me after another session of starvation dieting and pills that her weight problem was sneaking up on her again. "Gaining weight destroys my self-respect, increases frustration and brings morbid thoughts of death into my thinking day and night," she wrote. Obviously, this woman could not be beautiful in her state of mind.

It is not always this extreme. Overweight women generally have a lack of care about their clothes. Their hair and nails are not given the usual attention. They have a sluggish way about them. They have a wan, drawn look, and often rely heavily on make-up to hide poor skin condition. Their overall appearance is dull, unkempt.

Beauty can thrive only in a mental climate that is conducive to it. There is a close relationship between beauty and happiness. An interest in life and a desire to be attractive to the opposite sex brings a grace to movement, radiance to the skin, brightness to the eyes and an energetic step. I call it the posture of beauty.

This posture is not something you do for yourself as much as it is something you stop doing to yourself. If you think fat and think ugly you are depriving your face and body of the exuberant glow of youth. Stop doing this to yourself. Start now to think thin and think beauty.

If you think aches and age, you are depriving yourself of agility and ability. Stop doing this to yourself. Start now to think youth and think action.

If you have switched to proteins, you have good reason to switch your thinking too. Your bloodstream is continually bringing a fresh flow of proteins, amino acids, vitamins and minerals to every part of your body. Even if the switch was made only a few hours ago, you have every good reason to believe a change has started for a more beautiful you.

Stand erect. Look at yourself in a full-length mirror. Smile! Beauty smiles back. The real you is beginning to shine through. A new joy of dynamic living has begun for you.

How To Assist Nature To Make You Beautiful

Your beauty posture—mental and physical—can be given a real assist by the way you eat. Your high-protein diet has already begun the process of beauty-building, but there are other things you can do to accelerate the beauty process.

Shortage of nutrients in the body are not always quickly corrected when restored in the diet. Sometimes a bodily imbalance causes an inability to absorb certain nutrients from the food supplied. Proteins, vitamins and minerals are likely to restore that balance in time, but meanwhile you can help things along by providing the needed nutrient in concentrated quantities.

Vitamin concentrates and food supplements are available from drug stores, health food stores and direct from manufacturers. Natural, rather than synthetic vitamins, are the better of the two because of their being more readily absorbed by the body. Here are the areas these and supplement vitamins help.

Vitamin A. Brittle, dull hair is improved, and dandruff alleviated. Eyes are brighter, nails stronger, and noticeable improvements attained in skin condition.

Vitamin B. Irritability can be caused by a lack of this vitamin, and you cannot be beautiful with an ugly disposition. Nerves benefit from this vitamin.

Vitamin B1. Fatigue, depression, and stress take over when this vitamin is scarce. Use it to restore vim, vigor and joie de vivre.

Vitamin B2. Goes to work with Vitamin A and B to improve nerves and add youth to skin and eyes.

Vitamin B6. An aid to beauty sleep, good for the nerves, an excellent food for the skin and scalp.

Vitamin B12. A blood conditioner and thus a catalyst to the effective action of all vitamins and nutrients.

Niacin. Improves condition of gums and mouth. Helps the digestive process. A good skin and nerve food.

Paramino Binzoic Acid. Slows up graying of hair. Helps to improve natural hair color.

Inositol. Breaks down fats to their ingredient fatty acids and therefore improves contours. A good figure-restoring agent.

Chlorine. Appears to have a good effect on hair and skin.

Calcium Pantothenate. Good for the skin and the digestive system.

Bioten. Widespread benefits to the body through the restoration of glandular vitality. Noticeable effects on skin, hair, eyes.

Vitamin C. A boon to gums and teeth. Helps prevent infections, colds and their beauty-destroying symptoms. Good for certain allergies, too.

Vitamin D. Improves teeth and bones by helping body to utilize calcium.

Vitamin E. Known as the potency vitamin. Aid to vibrancy and vivacity.

Vitamin K. Helps your body's most vital organ—the liver. Your blood benefits too.

Calcium. Important to bones and teeth. When not supplied by the blood, bones and teeth actually give up their calcium to the blood to make up for the shortage.

Iodine. An aid to hormones. Removes sluggishness. Helps the skin and hair.

Iron. Good source of energy. An aid to the complexion, eyes, gums, teeth, hair and skin.

Phosphorus. Improves muscular response by aiding the functioning of nerves and brain.

Sulphur. Another useful ingredient for the luster of hair and the strength of nails.

The Way To Have a White and Bright Smile

The end to sweet and starchy foods and their replacement by savory protein-high dishes are now bringing a number of health and beauty dividends, an important one of which is a new and brighter smile.

Sugary food is the chief cause of tooth decay and periodontal (gum) disease rampant in 85 to 90 percent of otherwise healthy adults. Their contact with the teeth and gums can do even more harm than general nutritional deficiencies—a case of what you do eat interfering with beauty more than what you do not eat.

Chewy candy which is most likely to stick to the teeth is the chief culprit. Sugary drinks are bad, too. Substitute the healthful snacks listed in a later chapter for candy and sweets. Substitute low-calorie soft drinks for the sugared ones.

Nutritional imbalances can be corrected by liberal amounts of Vitamin A, B complex and C. Calcium supplements will help teeth. An old favorite—too old to know its source—is the use of strawberries as a toothpaste. Ask your grandmother. She did not know then that straw in the berries had just the right abrasiveness, that its Vitamin C was valuable to the gums, and that the acid in the berries removed stain from tooth enamel!

Ask your dentist to examine your teeth and gums for signs of diet deficiencies. Also have him show you how to improve your brushing technique to increase cleaning efficiency and gum stimulating advantages of this daily event.

Milk is rather high in carbohydrate and thus may be one of the foods that you will be cutting down on your high protein diet. In order to counteract this loss of an important calcium source, consider such calcium-high vegetables as kale, mustard greens, turnip greens and broccoli.

A good calcium supplement is available in the form of dried skim milk powder. There is also a very finely ground bone flour that can be used to thicken gravies and stews and add white to your smile.

How To Get a Peaches-and-Cream Complexion

The first improvement in beauty that protein will bring about will be reflected on the skin. The outer garment of the body is quick to betray malnutrition and mal-thinking. It is just as quick to portray wholesome food and wholesome thoughts.

Women are keenly aware of the importance of their skin to personal attractiveness. But they are less aware of the importance to the skin of a healthy body and a healthy mind. I have seen women sit helplessly by and watch their face get older and older, apparently resigned to the fact that the time in life had arrived when this step in aging was inevitable.

They do not suspect for a minute that this is a false or premature aging that can be halted and indeed reversed. You can imagine the effect on their personality and outlook on life when I show them how to bring back the youth and vitality they thought they had lost forever.

Then there are the women who think they can live on coffee, pills and cigarettes and enjoy a peaches-and-cream complexion. They are the ones who try every liquid cream and powder make-up on the market and wonder what is missing. I do not want you to think I am against cosmetics. They are fine, but they are not the whole story. Let me give you the simple steps to a complexion that is glowing with beauty. First, make the protein switch. Second, let go of the chocolates, pastries and sweets. Third, dwell on your blessings and be glad about life. Fourth, help nature to make you beautiful.

The first two steps you are now in the midst of. The third, you are resolving to take by improving your mental posture toward beauty, and there will be more valuable techniques to accomplish this later in this book. The fourth—help nature—I would like to elaborate on now.

Feed Your Skin the Nourishment It Needs

Assuming that you are helping nature with a high-protein diet which includes liberal amounts of high-vitamin and high-mineral content foods, and assuming that those who need to are taking vitamin and mineral supplements, there are still ways to feed your skin even more generous nourishment without partaking of a single calorie.

Remember how grandmother used crushed strawberries as an effective toothpaste? Well, she had a few more tricks up her sleeve, or I should say in her cupboard, and they work today just as they worked in her day.

Let us start with a face cleanser. Have you heard of olive oil, lanolin and glycerine? Equal parts. Put it on, take it off. See the difference?

How about a beauty mask of raw egg white? It works. It should; it is pure protein. The skin absorbs it readily and it is a shortcut to skin cell reinforcement.

There is a similar natural food remedy that is remarkably effective for just about every skin problem you can name. Chapping? Dissolve tapioca in hot water; make it a creamy mixture; rub in, rinse off. Blemishes? Equal parts of lanolin, glycerine and castor oil; blend the mixture over a mild heat; store in a covered glass jar in the refrigerator for regular use until pimples or other complexion blemishes disappear. Sun exposure? Plain apple cider vinegar. Wrinkle lines under the eyes? Apply moist tea bags for a spell. Other skin wrinkles on the face? Try rubbing castor oil into the wrinkled area.

To top off this menu for healthy skin, the phrase "peaches-and-cream" complexion was not the work of a poet but rather the work of a natural nutritionist: fresh peaches and cream, blended into a lotion and applied to the face, can actually bring about its namesake! When grandmother was young, she may have had her own private improvement on this one—blending strawberries and cucumbers into the peaches and cream for more dramatic results.

All of these natural aids work. Ask my 1,000 beautiful women. They are not meant to be a substitute for internal nutrition. Internal nutrition comes first, especially the B vitamins. These appear to play an important part in skin beauty.

Brown spots and brown areas can be due to B vitamin deficiency, as can redness and dryness. But there are many other causes of these symptoms.

Dryness is one of the most universal skin problems. It is prevalent in the days of summer sun and winter radiators. Too much sun and wind can rob the skin of the protective oil that prevents moisture from leaving the skin too rapidly. In spite of a healthy condition due to all the steps we have mentioned, a few hours of sun and wind can cause an acutely dry, rough and cracking condition. And a few weeks of steam heat can do the same. English women are famous for their complexions because of the moist climate and lack of central winter drying heat.

Natural oils can be restored by applications of lanolin, olive oil, castor oil, coconut oil or any of the oils that nature provides. Their names were legend among famous beauties of history, but many of these natural beauty aids have succumbed to less effective creams made of synthetic or soap products.

Sweet butter beaten with honey makes a fine food for the skin. Almond oil and honey has been from time immemorial a favorite skin lotion. There is no better moisturizer than water. A famous dermatologist was fond of saying that if there were no water he would have to invent it. In the Nordic countries, where most women have beautiful skin, it is their conviction that a mild soap should be used only with tepid, never hot, water.

There is so much to know about the skin, and it is so important to beauty that I am devoting an entire chapter to the many skin problems women are confronted with and how to cope with them naturally.

Beauty's Crowning Glory of Hair

The texture and luster of hair, in my opinion as a male, is a close second to skin as an important beauty feature in women. Clean, healthy hair has both texture and luster naturally. Every hair spray, shampoo, tint and restorer on the market strives to attain the perfection of nature. Unfortunately, more come close to the natural look in their advertising copy than in their actual performance.

Those products which use nature's foods, even if suspended or mixed with synthetics, are more likely to do a good job than those that are strictly chemical.

But the best of all possible jobs will be done by you. You are the sole feeder of your hair from the inside. The protein, vitamins and minerals you include on your daily diet will keep your hair's sheen and texture attractive to men, and the envy of women.

When you took steps to break away from starches and sugars, you took giant steps toward hair beauty. When you added vegetable oils to crisp green salads you made further progress. Women with excessively oily hair will find vegetable oils will help their condition while animal fats will aggravate it. Fur farmers in this country and Europe found that foxes' fur became much more valuable if linseed oil was added to their diet. The fur went from stringy and scrawny to shiny and shimmering.

If you have not been on a low-carbohydrate diet you have never seen the full, natural shade of your own hair. Before you pick one from a magazine or a bottle label, you might want to give your natural color a try.

Case History of the Natural Brunette Who Strayed

Jaquie L. was a plain brunette in her teens, a golden blonde when she married. She tried being a redhead after her first baby, realized it was out of tune for her, and was silver blonde when I saw her at age 35, and about 25 pounds overweight. When she began to take her natural shape, after a few weeks of high-protein dining, I convinced her she should stop trying to have her hair take attention away from the rest of her now shapely body. The result was one more natural beauty added to the dwindling ranks of the brunettes.

If your hair color is all yours, it can be genuinely attractive. But, I am not against helping nature. For instance, if you add the whites of two eggs to Castile shampoo and beat to a foam, you will be giving your hair a fine protein treat as you shampoo it. Massage the yolks into your hair and let stand a few minutes before rinsing and you bring protein right to the point where it is needed.

Nor am I against helping nature to bring out the color highlights in your hair. The juice of two lemons in slightly more water used as the final rinse and permitted to dry in the sun will bring out the golden highlights. Cider vinegar in the rinse water, followed by clear water, will do wonders for a brunette; and chamomile tea, brewed and mixed with a pint of water, used as a last rinse will accentuate the reds in your hair's spectrum.

Your hair is the frame for your beauty. It deserves your fondest attention and most fastidious care. But it is only the frame. The rest of you must be slender and attractive. In a hurry to get there? The next chapter tells you how to get there fast without starvation, will power or tears.

Review of Chapter Highlights

Begin to **feel** beautiful today. Hold yourself erect and let the natural joy for life radiate in your face. Choose vitamin or food supplements to strengthen your weak points. Select a natural food for your skin and begin daily or weekly facials. Restore natural beauty to your hair by feeding it right from the inside, as with vegetable oils on your salad, and from the outside with protein shampoos and lemon or vinegar rinses.

6

How To Lose Unwanted Pounds Fast

and for Good

The word *diet* is from the Greek *diaita* meaning a "manner of living" or "a way of life." It has somehow come to mean almost the opposite—a temporary way of eating. To diet really should continue to mean a permanent manner of discriminate eating.

You know how I feel about trying to lose weight on a diet, in its temporary sense. I think it is a useless exercise that is doomed to eventual failure. If you manage to stay on whatever diet you select until you reach your goal, congratulations. But if you are still at that goal a year later, I'll be amazed. The odds are in favor of your gaining back all you lost and possibly more.

By swapping proteins for carbohydrates you transform a fattening diet way of life to one that is non-fattening and which indeed will cause you to lose weight, albeit ever so gradually.

However, many overweight women are anxious for fast results and a gradual slimming over the years does not solve their problem *today*. This chapter is addressed to those who wish to lose weight fast. It shows you how to lose 10 to 15 pounds a month, and even more. It is not just another useless diet session which will end up like all the rest. This one is for keeps.

How To Start Your Unwanted Pounds Tumbling

I have good news for you. All of the principles that have applied in the foregoing chapters about easy slimming continue to apply now. In other words, it's easy to slim down fast. No major changes in your way of eating, no starvation and deprivation. Thanks to proteins, vitamins and minerals, you can truly enjoy eating well even on a serious weight loss program.

Kate Smith is reported to have once said that the world's most effective diet consists of exactly four words—"No more, thank you." It will be easier to say those words on a high protein way of life. Protein is filling and satisfying. Half a broiled chicken is considerably more filling than cottage cheese, and yet it has fewer carbohydrate calories. It is very much on the Petrie diet program, along with hundreds of other savory dishes.

To make your pounds begin to tumble faster you need to make some more substitutions of proteins for carbohydrates. You will use the same menus that you worked with at the end of Chapter 2. However, quantity is a factor too, and you will now utilize the point count system that has proved so popular with my now slender feminine friends.

Mrs. Burt Lancaster plans her famous husband's menu around protein. Fish and meat play a prominent role in keeping her husband in top physical shape, and gourmet dishes help satisfy the appetite's need for enjoyment.

However, occasionally any motion picture star, man or woman, must shed a few unwanted pounds fast to look right for the part. At these times, the high-protein diet is boosted even higher in protein. Also boosted is the high enjoyment value in order to compensate for quantity control.

There are two rules for quick weight loss:

1. Do not exceed 15 percent carbohydrate calories per day.
2. Do not exceed 1,000 protein and fat calories per day.

Protein can do wonders in slimming you gradually and keeping you slim, but they need your help to produce dramatic weight losses in short periods of time.

The helping hand you can lend proteins is the hand that reaches for second helpings. If you want to shift into high reducing gear, you must temporarily go easy on quantity.

Protein helps you to do this. Protein foods are long lasting in nourishment. Protein foods are delicious. You know you have eaten well when you have partaken of a steak smothered in mushrooms. It is nothing like most crash diets.

Furthermore, your basic need to enjoy eating is satisfied. You do not have that compulsion to raid the refrigerator that is often misunderstood for hunger.

Hunger is further reduced by the fact that you are supplying your body with all of the essential nutrients it needs. The appetite receives no distress signals like "Starving for amino acids down here in the leg muscles; rush supply." Every part of the body is being properly fed. The only shortage is in total heat and energy units called calories and that comes from your reserve supply called fat.

This fat is literally consumed by the body. It melts away as fast as an ounce an hour. I have seen women lose as much as 10 percent of their total weight in a month—20 pounds or 320 ounces. That's ten ounces a day or an average of one-half ounce every single waking hour for a month!

The Importance of Following Your Progress with a Chart

I am going to give you a very simple way to begin this fast rate of weight loss. I want to emphasize again that this is nothing like going on a diet. This is just a minor variation in your new way of life. But before I help you trigger this weight loss I want you to get ready to control it. Before you start a car you must know how and when to stop it.

To control your weight loss properly you need to "picture" or graph it on a chart. This is very simple, but nevertheless important. You can lose faster if the graph shows little change. You can lose more slowly if the graph shows too much change. You do this by cutting a few carbohydrate calories or adding them. Or you can cut down on portions or add a second portion of your favorite dish—pot roast, beef Stroganoff, etc.

The chart is made by using a piece of graph paper. If you do not have it, make one by drawing equally spaced horizontal and vertical lines. Let the vertical lines be labeled at the bottom with the date, starting at the left with today and inserting tomorrow's date next, etc. Let the horizontal lines be labeled with your weight, starting at the top with what you weigh today.

Now place a dot where the lefthand vertical line (today) intersects the top line (your present weight). Two or three times a week weigh yourself and put a dot where that day intersects the weight the scales read. Then draw a line from the previous dot. The resulting graph will reflect your progress at a glance.

This is an important control record. You can plot by a *dotted line* the downward course you want your weight to follow. Then your *solid line* of actual results can be compared to your goal on any given day.

How To Use a Diary to Control Carbohydrate Intake

There is another supplementary record you may wish to make. It is a more complete diary of your meal-to-meal, day-to-day, and week-to-week food intake. From it you can prove to yourself just how important it is to cut down on carbohydrate calories.

This weight loss diary requires a notebook. Each page is a week. On each page, the week is divided by horizontal lines into seven days with room at the bottom for totals. Three vertical lines divide the page sideways into four columns: breakfast, lunch, dinner, and in-between.

Each day enter your breakfast, lunch, and dinner, course by course, placing carbohydrate calories and non-carbohydrate calories alongside of each. Add them up at the end of each day, and at the bottom of the page, add up your weekly total.

Circle in blue those totals that remain below the proper quotas. Circle in red those totals that creep above the proper quotas.

Now by comparing blue circles to red circles you can see at a glance why your weight fell too fast or too slow. You have a full record of how weight loss depends on carbohydrate calories and on protein and fat calories. You will realize the impact that a few red carbohydrate circles can have on your scale. You will see the correlation week-by-week between food intake and weight loss.

How To Set Your Weight Loss Goal

How fat is fat? I have had lovely models wring their hands over a five-pound bulge. Other women with 30 pounds to spare admit reluctantly they could "drop a few."

Is there a right weight for women? Everybody is familiar with the age-height-weight tables found on penny scales. These are borrowed from statistics prepared by insurance companies. However, there appears to be a trend in average weights which makes these figures too low by about seven pounds for men and six pounds for women. Members of the faculty at Harvard's School of Public Health claim that, whereas insurance companies show a downward trend in weights for women, the last two decades show increasing weight when a full survey is taken.

For women in the eighteen to twenty-four age bracket, at 5'1", the conventional table calls for 112 pounds, but 117 would be closer to average. Similarly, in the thirty-five to forty-four age bracket, at height 5' 5", a reading of 135 pounds is about four pounds below the time norm.

The question arises: Is the normal or average weight of the populace an optimum or best weight? Nature has not provided a pattern or form by which we might judge the perfect body. But we can know the typical body. We can know its height, measurements, and weight. If the average American woman is overweight, then the typical body is overweight. There is no absolute standard by which to judge her.

I like to go on the assumption that the truth is somewhere between the insurance standards set up years ago and the present actual averages. Table 3 represents this compromise:

A fifty-five-year-old woman who suffered from hip and leg problems and who stood at 5' 7" in her stocking feet and 5' 9" in heels noted she weighed 202, just 35 pounds over the recommended

Height (In 2-inch heels)	Age 20-29	Age 30-39	Age 40-49	Age 50-59
5' 0"	115	125	131	133
5' 1"	119	128	134	136
5' 2"	122	131	137	139
5' 3"	125	134	140	143
5' 4"	128	137	144	147
5' 5"	132	140	147	151
5' 6"	136	144	151	155
5' 7"	139	146	155	159
5' 8"	143	151	159	163
5' 9"	147	155	163	167
5' 10"	151	159	168	172
5' 11"	156	164	173	177
6' 0"	160	169	178	183

Table 3

weight. She set a three-month goal; drew a progress chart with a dotted line slanting downward from 202 on May 22, her starting date, to 167 on August 22. On September 1 I received her chart in the mail. She had reached her goal on August 27, just five days late. The solid line ran very close to the dotted one.

There was a letter with her chart in which she wrote of how her hip and leg trouble had vanished. "I look and feel wonderful, and the best part is I am never hungry." She called the method the B's and C's of losing weight:

> No beans, bread, or beer
> No cake, cookies, or candy
> and P. S.—no potatoes, no sugar.

Lose Up to 1% of Your Weight Per Week

How steeply down should you chart your weight course? Should your graph plunge like a precipice or slope like a gentle hill? I like to hold the girls down to a loss of 1 percent of their weight a week. A 150-pounder should not lose more than one and one-half pounds a week. For a 200-pounder, the limit should be two pounds a week.

Even half of this top limit should be considered as adequate progress. In all likelihood, you will be losing weight in a fraction of the time you took to gain it.

Here are some tips about weighing yourself to assure accurate progress records. Many women avoid daily weigh-ins because the imperceptible daily changes have a tendency to be discouraging. They prefer weighing themselves every two or three days. On the other hand, others claim that relapses can be spotted quicker if weighing is on a daily basis. I do not think a system should be based on relapses, so I prefer "weighing in" once every two days, when a quarter- or half-pound change can be detected.

Keep your scale in the same spot. Stand on it always in the same erect position and the same degree of undress. Weigh in at the same time every day. These uniformities will serve to prevent variations in readings due to extraneous factors.

The scale is set. The chart is ready. Now we are ready to gird for action.

The 1,200-, 1,000-, and 800-Calorie Diets

Losing weight fast is a temporary condition. Cutting back on food to lose weight fast is a temporary condition. Is there a risk of gaining this weight back after the temporary cutback? The answer is no, providing you have already changed your permanent eating habits to the *high-protein, low-carbohydrate way.*

There are no big changes from the high-protein, low-carbohydrate "slow loss" to the high-protein, low-carbohydrate "fast loss." There is no change in the times you eat, or the types of food you eat. There is a slight change in how much you eat. When you go back to your former quantity, you will, of course, stop losing weight, but you will not gain any back. Were you to go back to former carbohydrates, too, the story would most certainly have a fat ending.

How much do you have to cut back in order to start that weight graph descending? This varies among women.

Case History of the Woman Who Hardly Moved

Mrs. G. R., aged twenty-three, was a comptometer operator in a large firm of accountants. She complained of headaches, backaches, and severe tension. Her weight: 302 pounds! She had been married for three years and had no children. Of these years, she said, "they have been trying." She lived within two blocks of her employment. Her husband delivered her to the door and picked her up at 5 P.M. She sat at her machine all day. When she got home she sat some more. She did light housework but hated it. She was unable to lose weight on an 800-calorie diet, or at best lost only one pound a month.

I was fascinated by her lack of energy and activity and I asked her to wear a pedometer for one week. She did so. At the end of the week the pedometer measured eight miles. It would have had to register 33 miles to show that she had burned up enough energy in one week to eliminate one pound; instead eight miles indicated approximately 875 caloric expenditure of a quarter of a pound.

She slept eight hours a night or a calorie expenditure of 400 a night or 2,800 calories a week, in sleep. Her approximate expenditure during one whole week in activities other than movement or sleeping were 1,200 calories or 8,400 a week. In the test week she spent 2,800 calories in sleep, 875 in movement, and 8,400 in sitting around—a total of 11,000 for the week. Her total energy output was approximately 1,500 a day. In order for her to lose two pounds a week, she would have to maintain a rigid diet of not more than 500 calories a day. As this was an impossible requirement, I persuaded her to increase her daily energy by four periods of fifteen minutes each of activities. I didn't care what she did, as long as she moved.

In the end I was able to have her lose weight on 900 calories a day. She has been reducing successfully since then.

Theoretically, weight loss should begin as soon as the body is burning more total calories than it is receiving. But there is a receiving department that most calorie-counting nutritionists neglect to consider. All receiving is not through the mouth. The lungs' intake of air each day weighs many times as much as the mouth's intake of food. The air wastes expelled also weigh more than the food wastes excreted, but metabolic differences and changes in the body can cause wide variations in both.

Water Weight in the Body

Water absorption by the body can take place through the lungs, skin and stomach. I have seen weight loss and weight gain in one day of several pounds due largely to water. Many obesity specialists win friends and influence weight-conscious people simply by dehydrating them in the first few days of treatment, usually with diuretic medicines.

Deceptive Body Changes

Even the eye can be fooled by temporary bodily changes. The stomach, contrary to what most people think, is not situated near the navel. It is quite a bit higher in the abdomen, toward the left side, tucked up under the diaphragm where it is protected by the rib cage. It is a kind of a pouch about ten inches long. Its diameter is the fooler. Empty, it collapses like a deflated balloon. Full—and it can hold as much as two quarts of food—it bulges like an inflated balloon, expanding upward and downward. Upwards into the lungs, where it makes breathing difficult, and downwards into the abdomen, where its rotundity can be readily observed by yourself and your admirers. Four to eight hours later the bulge can disappear. You look less paunchy, but you can weigh the same.

Total Calories and Carbohydrate Calories

The only sure, permanent way to weight loss today for you is to cut back sharply on *total calories* and on *carbohydrate calories*. One without the other will not work. If you cut back on carbohydrate calories to 200 but eat 3,000 calories total, you are headed to be a circus fat lady. If you cut back on total calories to 1,200, mostly all of them carbohydrates, you may not become a freak, but you will never win any beauty contests either.

That has been the heartbreak of diets all these years. Women starve themselves on melba toast, cottage cheese and carrot sticks, cutting back to 1,000 total calories, and wonder why they still weigh the same. They weigh the same because, although their total calories are within bounds, their carbohydrate calories are way out of line for losing weight.

If you want to lose weight fast, begin by cutting back to 1,020 protein and fat calories; 180 carbohydrate calories, for a total calorie count of 1,200.

If this does not lose weight fast enough, go to 850 protein and fat calories, 150 carbohydrate calories, for a total of 1,000.

If this does not lose weight fast enough, go to 680 protein and fat calories, 120 carbohydrate calories, for a total of 800.

Do not go any further than this, unless you are specifically advised to by your physician. It was recently established by a medical research worker that you can lose as much weight on 800 total calories a day as you can on a starvation diet. The astonishing findings came when the researchers studied overweight patients who followed a rigid, scientifically controlled reducing regimen for one to two months. Here is how it went:

Proof of 800-Calorie Diet Cutting Weight as Much as "Starvation" Diet

For the first two or three weeks, the patients were put on a high-protein, low-carbohydrate diet very similar to my 800-calorie limit. This was followed by five to thirteen days of rigid fasting, with only calorie-free fluids such as water, coffee and tea permitted. After this starvation period, the patients went back on the 800-calorie diet for the balance of the study.

During the rigid fasting period, weight loss was more rapid, but when the 800-calorie diet was resumed all of this extra weight loss was completely regained. In other words, they lost no more weight with the period of starvation than if they had continued right along on the 800-calorie diet. The reason for this is that the weight loss during starvation comes largely from the body's protein—essential structural material that is borrowed and must be restored. It is estimated that 65 percent of the weight loss on starvation diets is contributed by these hard-to-spare proteins. But on a low-calorie diet, only 3 percent of the weight loss comes from protein portions of the body, and 97 percent comes from body fat.

The moral is: Don't think you are being overconscientious by cutting below 800 calories. You are imposing on your body with no benefits by doing so. Settle for a loss of fat that will gain you years of life expectancy. Set 800 calories as the lowest you will go in restricting your intake. *It is low enough.* If it does not work, make a record of your carbohydrate intake, cut it down, and add proteins to keep your calorie total at 800. Now you are bound to lose, possibly faster than you need. Remember to ease up to 1,000 if your weight loss is more than 1 percent of your total weight per week.

The Point Count System

It is easier to count to 100 than it is to 1,000. Based on this simple fact, I have created a point count system for slimming the ladies that has proved quite popular, if for no reason other than it is easier to handle arithmetically.

If you let 10 calories equal 1 point, you have fewer figures to remember, fewer to count, fewer to total. And the process is effectively simplified.

In Table 4, you will find menu-building lists of suggested foods that have figures after each item. *They are not calories. They are points.* In Group A are carbohydrate-heavy foods that must be severely limited. In Group B are all the others. Based on the point system:

The 1,200-total calorie diet is a 120-point diet, with a maximum of 18 "A" points.

The 1,000-total calorie diet is a 100-point diet, with a maximum of 15 "A" points.

The 800-total calorie diet is an 80-point diet, with a maximum of 12 "A" points.

Under each of these point diets you maintain carbohydrates at the 15 percent level. It is not advisable to cut below this, because there is often a reaction known as ketosis. This is a form of acidosis. Mild cases can make a person feel queasy and "liverish." Some physicians recommend that excessively overweight persons, say 20 percent or more, stay above 250 carbohydrate calories and sometimes even 300 carbohydrate calories to begin with, and then reduce it later if no ketosis develops—another good reason why I always recommend that the family physician be consulted regularly when you are on a fast reducing schedule.

A typical menu for a day on each of three diets follows. The foods are selected from the menu list at the end of Chapter 3. Note that although totals increase in the three diets, the carbohydrate count remains at 15 percent.

Typical 80 Unit Day

Breakfast

4 oz. orange juice	4
1 poached egg on ½ sl. toast	11

Lunch

3 oz. canned salmon	15
Med. tomato stuffed with cottage cheese	6
Lettuce base with 5 asparagus sticks.	1

Dinner

4 oz. sliced roast beef	20
with natural gravy	0
1 c. fresh cauliflower	4
Tossed green salad	2
1 T. french dressing	8
2 fresh plums	4
1 Rye crisp	2
2 T. skim cottage cheese	3

Typical 100 Unit Day

Breakfast

½ c. strawberries	5
Grilled cheese 1 sl. bread	15

Lunch

Turkey salad 3 oz.	18
1 T. mayonnaise	10
Lettuce and tomato	2

Dinner

Medium lobster (6 oz. meat)	12
2 oz. drawn butter	10
1 c. oven baked broccoli with ¼ c. cheese sauce	11
Fresh peach	6

Late snack

2 soda crackers	3
2 T. Leiderkrantz	8

Typical 120 Unit Day

Breakfast

4 oz. tomato juice	2
2 eggs and 3 slices crisp bacon	26

Lunch

Chef salad made with base of lettuce, tomato & cucumber	4
2 oz. julienne turkey	12
1 slice julienne ham	4
1 slice julienne swiss cheese	9
1 T. french dressing	8

Dinner

4 oz. tomato soup	4
3 oz. sliced sirloin steak	23
6 stalks asparagus	1
Large tossed salad	3
Oil and vinegar dressing with 2 T. oil	6

Late snack

¾ c. loganberries	7
Medium pear sliced	6
Add 2 T. whipped cream	5

Table 4

Review of Chapter Highlights

Make your weight tumble faster with more protein for carbohydrate substitutions. Use a progress chart to control the process. There is no need to cut down to less than 800 calories. The point count system is easier to apply than calorie counting.

7

How To Work "Instant Youth" Miracles

As you lose weight, you lose years off your appearance and you feel younger. You actually regain youth. In this chapter I will help you to help nature make you young again. Instant, perpetual youth was what Ponce De Leon sought in the early 16th Century when he searched for the legendary fountain of youth. I have no such miraculous source, yet miracles do occur.

A forty-six-year-old mother told me that her own daughter did not recognize her when they met in front of a New York restaurant after only two months apart. A fifty-seven-year-old stenographer complained to me that men are whistling at her, something she had trouble with some thirty years before.

You know these miracles are possible. You have seen television and movie actresses appear year after year and decade after decade looking just as young as ever. Maybe you even have a friend or acquaintance who, despite her age, keeps that glow of youth and who seems to laugh at the years which make their unwanted mark on other women.

What do these women do? Is the answer hormones? Plastic surgery? Yoga? The world has seen perpetual youth sold in boxes, bottles and charms. It has been dispensed by traveling salesmen, books, department stores and medicine men. And it always will be. But it will not always provide the answer for you.

Premature aging is an effect that follows a cause. The cause can be quite different for one person than another. But remove that cause and you can reverse the aging process.

The foregoing took just a few seconds for me to write and less for you to read, but it is not easy to do and some women can never truly succeed at doing it. Yet I have helped more than 1,000 women to reverse the causes of their aging instantaneously!

Poor Diets Are the Youth Wreckers

What are the chief causes of premature aging? I point the finger at poor diet. Poor physical diet and poor mental diet. We are what we eat and we are what we think. The body must be well nourished and the soul must be well nourished.

The youth wreckers in our physical diet are the sweets and the starches and the refined and denatured foods. They are the negative foods that leave our body crying for vitamins, minerals and proteins, keys to physical youth.

The youth wreckers in our mental diet are the worries and the fears, the self-limitation and the pessimism. They are the negative attitudes that leave our soul crying for the joy of creative living and meaningful experience, keys to mental youth.

Women have come to me who have been through elaborate plastic surgery. They look weird close up. A face that has been worn by life's tribulations then "lifted" by plastic surgery is an unnatural face. Women who have had silicone injected into hollows in their faces or into breasts they wish to enlarge, a thriving practice especially in Mexico and Japan, are courting trouble—the same trouble that plagued women years ago who tried the same thing with paraffin. The result was often lumpy tumors.

You cannot eliminate the effects of the aging process and still permit the causes to erode away, physically or mentally. If you try to do this, it just does not come out right. You can always see through heavy make-up, and the heavier it is, the easier it is to see through. The more you try to hide the effects of poor physical diet or poor mental diet, the easier it is to "see through" the attempts.

Women live longer than men in most Western nations, but in the underdeveloped countries they live shorter lives than men. Women age faster than men in India, Vietnam, Cambodia, and Indonesia. Here the effects of malnutrition are compounded in a society that does not recognize the woman as the equal of a man. A diet of self-limitation and self-disrespect coupled with a diet largely devoid of nutrients can work miracles of aging.

What about hard work? Hard work requires a diet richer in nutrients, but hard work in itself is not a youth wrecker, contrary to what many may think. The old adage that hard work never killed anyone is still true, and I would like to add that it never made anyone look old either. I am not speaking about severe, prolonged exertion beyond one's physical endurance. This is indeed aging and even killing. But strenuous work—physical or mental—to which one has grown accustomed can indeed promote youthfulness and longevity.

Food for the Mind

The new slimming fare that you are now on satisfies the body's need for nutrients and ends youth wrecker No. 1—body deficiency. But how do you improve your mental fare?

Geriatric experts now state that length of life beyond the normal expectancy is influenced by alertness of the mind. Certainly an active mind is a sign of youth, but which comes first, the active mind or the youthful mind? The answer is vital if we are to lick youth wrecker No. 2—poor mental diet.

I believe that an active mind comes as a natural follow-up of removing this youth wrecker No. 2. Activating the mind in a climate of negative attitudes is as futile as activating the body as a means to good nutrition. But remove negative attitudes and behold a miracle!

So here is the key: Wholesome attitudes permit an active mind and release the powers of youth. It works. It begins instantaneously. Ask my 1,000 women clients.

As you see, there is no fixed quota for breakfast, lunch or dinner. You are free to eat larger or smaller breakfasts just as you do now. You can even spurt up the meals differently if that will cause the least change from your present way of life. Remember, the less the change in this way, the easier it is to stay off the weight-gain treadmill.

Get ready for that new wardrobe. The weight you lose in the days ahead are gone forever. When you go back to your full high-protein diet, you will not go back to your full measure. You will stop losing, but you will stay thin.

THE POINT COUNT FAST REDUCING DIETS

Pick foods from Group A and Group B. Stay within the limits shown on each, depending on whether you are on the 80, 100, or 120 point diet.

GROUP A

Juices (4 oz.)

Blackberry	3
Red currant	4
Grapefruit	4
Loganberry	4
Orange	4
Pineapple	5
Raspberry	4
Sauerkraut	1
Tomato	1

Fruit

Cantaloupe ½ med.	5
Strawberries ½ c.	5
Raspberries ½ c.	5
Tangerine 1 med.	2
Orange 1 med.	6
Grapefruit ½ med.	5
Pineapple 4 oz.	6
Plums 2 med.	4
Blackberries ½ c.	5
Apple 1 med.	7
Apricot 2 med.	6
Blueberries ½ c.	6
Cherries 7	5
Grapes 3 oz.	6
Loganberries ½ c.	7
Nectarine 2 med.	7
Peach 1 med.	6
Pear 1 med.	6
Rhubarb 1 c.	2
Watermelon 4 oz.	5

Flours

Cornmeal wht. 7 yell. ¼ c.	12
Cornstarch 1 T.	4
Gluten ¼ c.	13

Soybean ¼ c.	7
Self-rising ¼ c.	11

Yeast

Bakers dried 1 T.	5
Brewers dried 1 T.	5
Compressed moist 1 cake	2
Dried ½ cake	5

Vegetables

Asparagus 6 stk.	1
Bamboo shoots ½ c.	1
Broccoli 1 c.	5
Cabbage 1 c.	2
Cauliflower 1 c.	4
Celery 2 stk.	1
Cucumber ½ m.	1
Endive 5 leaves	1
Fennel 1 c.	1
Lettuce 4 leaves	1
Greens 1 c.	2
Radishes 5 med.	1
Romaine ½ head	2
Squash ½ c.	2
Tomato 1 med.	2
Watercress 10 pc.	1
Mushrooms 16 lg.	1
Pepper (green) 1 med.	3

Bread & Crackers

Parker house roll 1 m.	5
Toast or bread 1 sl.	6
Cream crackers 2 med.	4
Soda crackers 2 med.	3
Rye Krisp 1	2
Water crackers 1	3

Table 5

Group A Maximum Units				Vegetables	4	5	6
	80	100	120	Flour, yeast bread & crackers	3	4	5
Juices & fruits	5	6	7	Total	12	15	18

Group B

Fish c—cooked r—raw 4 oz.

Anchovies	17	Sturgeon smoked	14
Bass (black) r	10	Swordfish (broiled)	18
Carp r	9	Trout (steamed)	11
Caviar r	25	Turbot r	19
Clams r	8	Tuna canned	19
Codfish r	5	White fish (broiled)	15
Crab c	8		
Croaker c	10	*Meats*	
Eels r	16	Poultry (cooked) 3 oz.	
Finnan haddie c	10	Chicken	18
Flounder r	6	Turkey	18
Frogs' legs (4)	4	Duck	18
Haddock (broiled)	10	Veal chop 1	15
Halibut (broiled)	12	Lamb (leg)	26
Herring r	14	Liver, beef	17
Herring can. in tomato s.	17	Liver, calf	16
Herring kippered	20	Liver, pork	15
Lobster (broiled)	8	Bologna 2 sl. ⅛" thick	4
Mackerel r	18	Frankfurter 1	10
Mullett r	12	Head cheese 1 sl. 1/16" thick	7
Oysters 4	8	Luncheon meat 2 1/16" thick	9
Perch (broiled)	20	Sausage 2 links	8
Pike r	8	Liver sausage 2 sl. 1/16" thick	5
Pompano r	16	Salami 2 sl. 1/16" thick	11
Porgy r	9	Boiled ham 1 sl. ⅛" thick	4
Red snapper r	9	Fresh ham 2 sl. ⅛" thick	14
Salmon smoked	17	Hamburgers 1¼" thick	14
Sardines canned in oil	20	Corned beef hash 3 oz.	13
Sardines canned in tomato	17	Heart 3 oz.	15
Scallops r	7	Round pot roast 30 oz.	18
Shad (broiled)	21	Rib roast 3 oz.	24
Shrimp c	8	Club steak 3 oz.	19
Sole r	8	Porterhouse steak 3 oz.	28
		Sirloin steak 3 oz.	23

Table 5 (Continued)

GROUP B

Soups

Bouillon	4 oz.	1	Salmon	3 oz.	15
Consommé	4 oz.	4	Egg (2)		16
Cream of asparagus	4 oz.	11			
Cream of celery	4 oz.	11	ADD FOR 1 T DRESSING		
Cream of mushroom	4 oz.	10	French		8
Cream of tomato	4 oz.	11	Mayonnaise		10
Split pea	4 oz.	10	Roquefort		12
Tomato	4 oz.	4	Thousand Island		8
Vegetable	4 oz.	5	Oil		10
			Vinegar or lemon		0

Eggs

1 egg	8
add for 1 t. butter, margarine or bacon fat	3
add for	
ham 1 sl. ⅛" thick	4
Sausage 1 link	4
Bologna 2 sl.	4
Bacon 2 sl.	7
Bacon Canadian 2 sl.	6

Dairy

Milk whole 2 oz.	4
Milk skimmed ½ c.	4
Milk skimmed dried 1 T.	2
Milk whole dried 1 T.	3
Buttermilk ½ c.	4
Coffee cream 1 T.	3
Whipped cream 2 T.	5

Cheeses

Cream 1 T.	8
Cheddar 1 cube	8
American 1 sl.	9
Cottage 2 T.	4
Cottage (skim) 2 T.	3
Liederkranz 1 T.	4
Swiss ⅛" sl.	9
Velveeta ⅛" sl.	6
Münster 1 oz.	10
Parmesan 2 T.	4

Note

These are additions to crackers —Count the unit for crackers plus the unit count below.

1 oz. cheese	10
1 oz. cottage cheese	4
1 oz. sardines	4
1 oz. salmon	5
1 oz. tuna	4
1 oz. egg salad	5
1 oz. chopped liver	5
1 oz. smoked salmon	4

Salads

Tuna	3 oz.	10
Chicken	3 oz.	18
Turkey	3 oz.	18
Lobster	3 oz.	8

Sauces

Béchamel 2 T.	5
Brown 2 T.	4

Table 5 (continued)

Sauces (*cont.*)

Cheese ½ c.	6	Soy 2 T.	2
Cranberry 2 T.	7	Tartar 1 T.	10
Cream ¼ c.	10	Tomato ¼ c.	5
Curry ⅓ c.	11		
Drawn butter ¼ c.	10		

Group B

Maximum Units

80	100	120
68	85	102

Hard sauce 2 T.	19
Hollandaise 2 T.	13
Lemon (with egg)	11

Table 5 (continued)

There may be a few self-disciplined weeks ahead but your new lovely silhouette will be yours for keeps. Yours, too, will be a new youth, and a healthy, energetic life.

The power of the mind over the body is a never-ending source of wonder. Thoughts and attitudes can control the heart beat, the rate of growth, the appearance of the body. Thoughts and attitudes can make us robust or weaken our resistance to disease. Thoughts and attitudes can spur us to a successful life or crush us under a paralyzing burden of apparent obstacles.

If you could control your thoughts, wouldn't you prefer to think confidence than worry? If you are confident, can't you just picture yourself youthful and erect, energetic and creative? If you are fearful, your self-portrait is of a person stooped with the burdens of life, wracked with indecision and literally paralyzed from all creative action. If you could control your thoughts, you would certainly pick the confident you.

Case History of the Woman Who Courted Failure

Mrs. D. M. wrote to me from Portland, Oregon, asking for an appointment. She said, "I am desperate. I can't seem to lose weight, but then again I doubt my ability to do anything well." We arranged an appointment and I found her to be one of the many who had been conditioned to be negative about themselves.

She had dieted unsuccessfully all of her life and just like the insomniac who goes to bed not expecting to sleep, she started each of her diets not expecting to succeed. She was full of inhibitions and feelings of inadequacy. She told me she had been attending psychiatric therapy on and off for the last seven years but there, too, she found herself an inadequate patient.

She had been partially convinced that the need to eat was a repressed sexual outlet. But, as she said, "If I now have insight to my problem, why can't I control my appetite?"

As she was only to stay in New York five days, I saw her every day, sometimes as long as two hours each period. I believe I convinced her to start again as from now, to consider her food logically in terms of calories, carbohydrates and the size of her waistline. I pointed out to her that she had lost weight. Surely that was a period of success. I gave her a program to follow and a letter to her physician back home. I talked to her about conditioning and how she now has to unlearn all of her old habits. We talked about her assets and not her liabilities.

We must have been successful. Six months later I received another letter and she said, "I am sorry I didn't do this ten years ago when I started putting on weight; it is the first time in my whole life that I felt confident. I am beginning to know what to do and how to do it. Thank you again so very, very much for putting me on the road to becoming the person I have always wanted to be."

How To Make Your Reflexes Work for Your Benefit

Up until now you have not been able to control your thoughts. Your thoughts are habit. If you have gone to bed being jealous of your sister, you wake up still jealous of your sister. If you are afraid to speak in public on Monday, you are the same way Tuesday. You do not reason it out each time. You accept your present thoughts.

However, many of these thoughts are out of style, obsolete, no longer true. Yet they persist. An angry father may turn to a ten-year-old girl who just knocked over a vase and explode with, "You clumsy brat. You're too stupid to even look where you're going!" It must be true, because there are the broken pieces of the vase in front of her. She accepts that image of herself. She wakes up with it the next day. It drifts into her subconscious, where it is soon consciously forgotten but where it remains as her official conditioner, along with many other impressions of herself that follow from later experiences.

We all have these conditioned reflexes. Many of us are conditioned to spring into confident action. Others of us are conditioned to sink into fearful withdrawal. Deep in our subconscious we create a self-image of youthful ability or a self-image of senile incapability.

What we don't know is: we *can* recondition our reflexes. That's right. We can wipe the slate clean of any reflex we don't want, and reprogram ourselves with a new reflex in its place. And the process does not take years. It takes minutes.

How To Recondition Yourself To Let Youth in the Easy Way

Will you do a simple mental exercise right now? It can be a turning point in your life. It will take only sixty seconds. Here is what I want you to do. When I say "Now!" I want you to put this book down, close your eyes and visualize the following: You see two roads. Down the left road you see yourself afraid, unhappy, old. On the right road you see yourself confident, happy, young. It is all very clear; you do not want your life to be like you see it on the left hand road, so you see yourself choosing the right hand road and starting on your way. Put the book down. Now!

You have just done something in your thoughts that is actually very real and alive. Thoughts have a way of bringing themselves to come about, especially when they are thoughts about yourself.

My 1,000 women clients have grown actually young by sitting in a chair, relaxing their bodies, and then visualizing properly. Their visual images of disliking cake and potatoes have brought about a dislike for those fattening foods. Their visual images of themselves enjoying coq au vin and crisp salad have enhanced their enjoyment of those healthful foods.

Their images of abandoning old patterns of self-pity and remorse and adopting new patterns of self-appreciation and expectation have brought about new patterns of youthful accomplishment and a real new look in their persons.

I am going to give you a few of these mental exercises to do in a relaxed state. They are all aimed at removing youth inhibitors that lurk in our own self-images. The better relaxed you are, the better they will work. Do them whenever you have a moment. Perhaps when you put your feet on the floor on awakening in the morning, or before you go to bed, or after a meal. Always be comfortable and free of distractions. Quiet the mind. Erase thoughts as fast as they creep in. Then, when the mind is clear, start visualizing.

Let me give you a tip. The mind does not want to be changed. It likes the way it is. Habits are habits, to the mind as well as to the body. So, your mind may trick you into forgetting to do these visual exercises. It may say, "Don't waste time," or "There's plenty of time tomorrow." Just remember it's *your* youth waiting to be recaptured, just a few conditioned reflexes away.

Here are three more exercises of the imagination that will help recondition your attitudes to let youth in:

Reconditioning Exercise No. 1

Sit in a comfortable chair. Feel yourself go limp. You are so relaxed that you have no desire to move. Your mind is serene. You enjoy this blissful state. Now give yourself instructions as follows, but be sure you mean them, because instructions given to oneself in this relaxed state are very powerful: *I will have a keen interest in new activities. I know that everything new I do is an expression of my youth. I will have a keen interest in new activities.* (Repeat this six times.)

Reconditioning Exercise No. 2

Be seated comfortably. Relax thoroughly. Feel your limbs get heavy as deep relaxation comes over your entire body. Imitate a rag doll. Go completely limp. The only thing holding you is the chair. Pretend you are unconscious. If your arm was lifted it would fall back like a dead weight. Breathe deeply and regularly as you do when you are asleep. Remove tension from your face muscles. Let your head drop slightly. Now relax your mind. Make believe you are at the movies, alone. The screen is empty. Now a full-length image of you comes on the screen. As you watch this picture of you, changes occur. You look younger and more beautiful. Your weight goes down and you look slim and youthful. You wear a white sheath dress. There is a close-up of your face. Your skin is perfect. It is clean, tight and firm. Your hair is lustrous and attractive. You see yourself as you will be. You know that this is your goal and that you are on the way to attaining it.

Reconditioning Exercise No. 3

Stand in front of a full-length mirror. Know what you are like now. Note that your posture is not so good as it might be. There are lines on your face. Your stomach is large and seems to bloat the rest of you. Now stand erect, belly in. Use your hands to smooth the wrinkles. See yourself young again. Accept the fact that you can look and feel young again. Accept this as reality. Know that this book and its methods work, that women everywhere have been helped, that you are being helped right this minute. You see how step-by-step your age lines will diminish, you will become deflated and more slender. You decide to become vain. You know that to say "I can't" will keep you as you are. So you close the exercise with the ultimate in vanity—you repeat: *I am the most beautiful woman in the world.*

Case History of the Tense School Teacher Who Relaxed

Miss L. B. was a teacher in an elementary school. As a child she was overweight; by the time she had reached sixteen she weighed 160 pounds. By twenty she was 175 pounds and now at twenty-nine she struggled with 155 pounds. Her right weight should have been approximately 130, but she said, "I'm too nervous, and whenever I get nervous I eat."

I attempted three separate diets with Miss L. B. without success. She was, as she said, too nervous.

I decided to use a system of hypnosis called progressive relaxation. Miss L. B. was both reluctant and fearful. I explained to her that progressive relaxation would allow us to accomplish two things. First it would relieve her of nervous tensions and secondly would allow me to offer post-hypnotic instruction that would lessen her appetite and in fact would cause her to have no particular appetite for starches and sweets. I had used this system over a period of twelve years with literally hundreds of people, and found it to be amazingly successful. And so it was in the case of Miss L. B. She was a good subject. I taught her how to relax herself and to give herself suggestions that would fortify her resolve and take the load off her will power.

How To Make the Image of the Youthful You

If there were such a thing as an instant-youth pill that you could swallow, how would you look? Do you have a clear-cut idea of what ten years off your life means? What does change when age creeps over you and can you reverse the process in your mind's eye?

The first visit after a reconditioning session, I see changes in women. I see a new alertness in their eyes, a vibrance in their manner, a zip in their motion. True, they start to take more interest in their coiffure, cosmetics and clothes, but those are the superstructure. I am interested in a strong foundation of youth first.

Can you see yourself in your late teens or early twenties? Early

adulthood is the youthful image. It is the image you need to cultivate about yourself even if you are in your fifties. Women who know
the secrets of youth, be it through yoga—and I will have a word
about that technique in a minute—or through visual exercises, look
twenty years younger than their calendar years. The image of you as
a young adult is the very person inside you right now trying to get
out.

I asked Mrs. K., a young widow who never fully recovered from
the loss of her husband in combat, just how she managed to throw
off the yoke of self-pity and its aging effect so dramatically. What
did she use as her self-image? She replied that she went back to her
college days before she met her husband. She used a photograph of
herself to assist the reconditioning process. She remembered the fun
she had had during the year the picture was taken. She found she
was able to recapture the feeling of expectation of falling in love
again.

Can there be any doubt that this mental turnabout, this rejuvenation of the spirit, can cause a rejuvenation in appearance? Believe
me, it works like the law of gravity. I used the word miracle before.
I use it again. I have seen miraculous transformations as women fed
their bodies with high protein nourishment and nourished their
souls with positive images.

The reconditioning exercises you will do all involve programming
your subconscious to a youthful pattern. Since it is your subconscious that controls the functioning processes of the body, it can
make you young or it can make you old. You need to think young to
be young. You need to think younger than you think now to look and
feel younger than you do now. You can accomplish this consciously
over a long period of practice. But you can do it easier and faster
through the subconscious.

The hardest time I have had with my 1,000 women is to get them
to believe they can be slim, youthful and attractive. In the reconditioning exercise using the motion picture screen, many could not see
the screen, or if they did see the screen, they could not see themselves change in appearance.

This lack of self-confidence is the greatest obstacle. To have no
confidence in one's innate youthfulness and attractiveness can perpetuate age and unattractiveness.

A woman comes into my office. She looks about fifty. I put her on
the scale. She weighs 230 pounds. I make out her record card. She

admits to forty-one. She says she "would do anything to lose." She begins to lose. She is happy beyond words. I say she is going to weigh 136 soon. But at 175 pounds she slows up. She has apparently lost interest. She is no longer obese. She is passable. She always knew she could be passable. Never a beauty, but certainly passable.

I know differently. I can see her weighing 136. I can even see her underweight. She cannot see herself weighing 136. It does not matter how I see her; it is how she sees herself that counts.

A generation ago, forty-year-old women looked much older. The subconscious has adapted itself to this image. It takes movie stars a great deal of effort to recondition themselves to understand how youthful they can really look at their age. Seeing miracles happen around them helps build their own confidence.

Now, I don't blame a stout matron-like woman for having absolutely no confidence in her ever looking like she did when the wolf-calls rang loud and clear. If such a woman were to try to recondition herself to have confidence in attaining her former sylph-like self, she could build up quite an internal conflict, better known as a neurosis.

How can you have confidence in a miracle? You can't. That is, unless you see it happen again and again before your eyes, or hear about it with your ears. Few who travel to Lourdes disbelieving in a cure, ever get one. But those who *know* what has transpired with others before them expect a cure, and quite often it comes.

That is why I am very happy to receive before-and-after pictures of my clients. I put them on the wall. I show them continuously. They are miracles caught by the camera for posterity.

When the stout matron-like woman sees these pictures and hears about some of the case histories, the defeatist attitude begins to fade—a glimmer of hope begins. She begins to realize that the impossible is, after all, possible. She is in the right place. And it can happen to her.

You have the right book right now in your hands. And it can happen to you. I know that you can look years younger in just a matter of days.

I see the image of you that you must see, too. It may not be an image of a show-stopping beauty, but it is an image of a smart, well-groomed and radiant person. She has clear skin, a natural radiance, an alert awareness. Her trim figure moves gracefully as she expresses exuberance, enthusiasm, and energy. It is the image of you that you are becoming.

Yoga and Other Paths

There are a number of ways to discipline yourself to become young. Remember this: it took anxieties to produce age lines and wrinkles, many years of them. You must be willing to work at being young.

One very popular discipline is yoga. Many women whom I know have tried yoga. I have seen some remarkable results.

Hatha yoga is that form of the ancient Indian discipline so popular in the West today. The Sanskrit word "yoga" means "union" and is related to the English word "yoke." It implies a joining together of the outer self to the inner self—the physical with the spiritual. Hatha yoga is used primarily as exercise. It is similar to the stretching and relaxation of animals. It can be done by persons of all ages. Its body postures are done slowly, with the mind concentrating on different parts of the body, and with accompanying breathing. Very beneficial are the upside-down postures that reverse the pull of gravity on the internal organs. These include the shoulder stand, done by raising your feet until your weight rests on your head, shoulders and upper arms. The "plough" is similar except that the legs continue back until they touch the floor behind your head. Other types of yoga exercises include sitting crosslegged, imitating the cobra, swan and other graceful creatures. Each position is held for a while and there is a brief rest between postures. For more details, consult Indra Devi's excellent treatise on the subject.[1]

To the Japanese, gardening is one of the fine arts. To plan and carry to fruition a garden of one's own can be a joy and satisfaction, as well as fun and exercise. Every part of the body is flexed and stretched as a dancer's, and with no boring calisthenics. Spending long hours outdoors, breathing deeply, using the body—these are all aids to keeping young. The enthusiasm for creating a spot of beauty that can be shared by others is the enthusiasm of creative youth.

It is no secret that those who work with young people remain younger than their contemporaries who seek companionship among their own or older age groups; to work with the young, in whatever field, gives one the energy, open-mindedness, zest for living, flexi-

---

[1] Indra Devi, *Yoga for Americans* (Englewood Cliffs, N.J.: Prentice Hall, Inc., 1959).

bility, freshness of youth. It rubs off on you. No matter what your age, you can begin today to serve youth. Grandparents grow young playing with grandchildren. You can read to a blind child, donate your time to a cooperative nursery, work in a settlement house or any one of dozens of groups that assist youth. It may lead to a new career, or it may not, but it can mean a new and more youthful you.

Activity Makes Us Young

The young can be active. Everybody knows this. But how few know the active can be young. There is something about work that titillates the metabolic processes. Work that we hate can bow us to the ground. Work that we love can send us soaring.

"I wake up tired." This is the song of the bored and the aging. Even women in their thirties with all the labor-saving devices of this electrical age can hardly find energy to get through the day. The reason is that housework is boring. Women used to be able to chat with their neighbors while they did their chores, but now suburbia has done away with even that. Housework is lonely and boring.

The cemeteries are full of women who literally faded away behind a vacuum cleaner and dishwasher. Their lives closed in on them when they got deeper and deeper in the rut of uncreative housekeeping, until they became so deep they could no longer see the main purposes of existence for which housekeeping is but supportive service. When life's purpose disappears from view, aging begins. And it can come on fast.

Housework must be done. But there is much more that must be done. You must write, or paint, or sell, or type, or sail, or ride, or play cards. Women who keep busy, keep young.

What is there about activity that keeps us young? It is not the physical exercise, because mental activity will do just as well. It appears to be the interest, the challenge, and the chase. These are what keep us eager and wide-eyed in our youth. These are what will keep away the sagging and the shadows later.

People who start a new life, turn young again. To start a new life you do not have to make decisions about the path ahead; all you have to do is decide not to stay on the path you are on. The moment you make that decision you will start the juices in your body flowing.

"I give this up. I start anew." Say this to yourself right now. Look in the mirror and say it again and again. Nature abhors a vacuum. As you shut out the past, the future will appear.

Don't forget it. Let it in. Accept new opportunities as they appear. Talk to new people as they come into your life. Try new foods—high-protein foods, of course, bursting with vitamins and minerals. Go to new places, enjoy new hobbies, play new games.

The first step is to relax. Do the reconditioning exercises in a thoroughly relaxed state. Do them every day for one week. It is a small investment of time for the years of youth you will be on your way to gaining.

Review of Chapter Highlights

Reverse your aging process by eliminating worries and fear from your mental diet. Substitute wholesome, positive, confident attitudes. Become active and release the powers of creative youth within you. Use the mental exercises starting on page 85 to make the changes stick. Visualize how you look slender and more youthful. Hold that image of yourself in mind as you do a yoga exercise, work in the garden, or some other refreshing recreation activity.

8

How To Enjoy a "Pounds Lost Weekend"
Right in Your Own Home

How would you like to visit a health spa for a weekend of weight loss and youth gain, but right in your own home? I can guarantee you will never forget it and it will give you a giant headstart on your reducing program. No travel or resort costs, but you will get all the advantages of a trip to a "milk farm" or reducing camp.

It is a fun weekend. It is a weekend devoted to *you*. You will pamper yourself from Friday afternoon to Monday morning! You will cater to your every beauty and health need. You will eat well but you will lose weight, probably five pounds in the two days plus. You will look five years younger and feel ten years younger. And you will have such a good time you will want to do it again soon.

If you are single or live alone, you are ready to prepare for the adventure. If you have a family, you had best discuss your intentions with them. Explain how you want a weekend for yourself. It does not mean that you love them any less. In fact, you want to beautify yourself for them. But to do it, it may mean hours to yourself, and even meals alone. Challenge them to let you try it so that all can see the transformation it brings about.

Many women who have tried and tried and tried finally reach that point where they just do not feel like trying any more. They have worked and struggled to lose weight and have gotten nowhere. Now they are discouraged, ready to give up. You can guess the rest of that story, or maybe you know it from personal experience. Another round of sublimation of the emotions through food is about to get under way. And it will lead inevitably to another crisis either in health, family life, or emotions, another fall into the depths of frustration, sheer misery and despair.

YOUR WEEKEND SHOPPING LIST

1 bottle dry sherry

1 squab or 1 guinea hen
6 oz. chopped sirloin

6 oz. fillet of flounder, fresh or frozen

6 stalks asparagus	onions
1 bunch broccoli	radishes
2 cucumbers	strawberries (in season)
1 grapefruit	3 tomatoes
4 lemons	watercress
1 head lettuce	
1 doz. eggs	8 oz. pkg. swiss cheese
coffee for perc. or drip	8 oz. grated parmesan cheese
tea bags	¼ lb. cheddar cheese
skim dry milk	1 pkg. cream cheese
½ pt. cream	8 oz. cottage cheese
1 c. frozen lemonade	
1 pkg. D-Zerta	cayenne worcestershire sauce
1 box soya crackers	dry mustard vinegar

Optional items

garlic cloves   salad oil
paprika
1 pr. cotton gloves, large size   thyme
2 oz. oil of sweet almonds
" " cocoa butter
3 oz. lanolin
1 box alum
  almond oil
  mineral oil
  castor oil
  cocoanut oil
½ lb. castile soap
  ethyl alcohol

Figure 8-1

The weekend ahead is an uplifting affair. It will boost your morale, lower your weight, improve your looks, heighten your zest for life, renew your vigor and send you forth on Monday morning a brand-new, younger and more attractive person.

An impossible miracle, you say? You are right—a miracle, yes, but impossible, no. I have seen these weekend transformations. I should be blasé about them by now. But I am always as surprised and delighted as I was the Monday I saw my first client sweep into the office after a "pounds lost weekend." Today I still shake my head in astonishment, a thousand "weekends" later.

Are you ready to experience what may prove to be the happiest weekend of your life? There is no suitcase to pack. Just bring this book, for through it I will take you by the hand and instruct you step by step. It is now Friday afternoon. Your weekend has begun.

First Stop: The Supermarket

You are going to need some special ingredients to enjoy this weekend. They are all obtainable at your local food stores, drug store, etc. You may already have most of them at home. It is best to prepare now, though. Do your weekend shopping Friday afternoon so that all of your errands are finished and you can devote your full time to yourself.

Figure 8-1 is a list of what you will need in the way of food items and beauty aids. All quantities are for one person—yourself.

When I give this shopping list to a woman embarking on this weekend, there is usually a raised eyebrow or two. "Mr. Petrie, I question whether this weekend is going to add up to all you have said it will," complained one thirty-two-year-old 153-pound brunette. When I saw her three days later she was a 148-pound blonde and looked twenty-five.

A plain shopping list can yield some fancy living. Watch and see.

Start by Relaxing Your Cares Away

The moment you get home and are in the privacy of your weekend spa quarters, open the bottle of dry sherry and have a small wine glass full of this relaxing tonic. When you fill the glass, put the bottle away and out of sight. Sit in a comfortable chair and sip it slowly. Cup the glass in your hand and inhale its bouquet. Savour the flavor as you sip. Now take the squab or guinea hen, frozen or fresh, and put it in the oven to roast. It will be ready in 45 minutes to an hour and 15 minutes.

You are still geared to the week-day rush. Your mind is still working at a fast pace. You feel jumpy sitting still. Even the soothing effect of the wine has not been able to relax you fully. Tension causes overeating. You owe it to yourself to simmer down. Here is an easy way to do it.

Sit in a straight back comfortable chair. Take your shoes off. Do not lie on your bed, as this method is so effective you can easily fall asleep and we are not ready for that yet. Now place your hands on your knees and close your eyes. Take a deep breath. Exhale. Take a second deep breath, let your hands drop to your sides and as you exhale let your head sag to your chest. Then let the following thoughts flow through your mind. (You may have to read this paragraph two or three times in order to know the procedure, but then it will come easily and naturally to you.)

> *I am very comfortable. . . . I am sitting limply. . . . I am breathing slowly and regularly as if asleep. . . . I am getting more comfortable and relaxed with every breath I take. . . . I begin to feel a sensation of heaviness. . . . I know this heaviness to be a relaxed feeling. . . . My feet are becoming heavier and heavier. . . . The soles of my feet are relaxed, my toes are heavy and relaxed. . . . The heaviness creeps up into my ankles, my legs, my thighs. . . . My whole body feels heavier and heavier. . . . It is pleasant and comfortable. . . . My chest, my arms, my neck . . . now my whole body feels heavy and relaxed. . . . I can deepen this relaxation by becoming more aware of the heaviness. Heavier, heavier, heavier . . . my lower jaw relaxes and my mouth opens slightly. . . . My eyelids are so heavy I can hardly keep them open. . . . Now my eyes close. . . . I see the darkness. It is grayish black. . . . My mind is empty of thought. . . . I am doing nothing. . . . I am now thoroughly relaxed. . . . I will enjoy this state for a few minutes. . . . Now, before I arouse myself, I know I will feel recharged and full of energy. . . . I visualize a thinner and a younger me. . . . Now I lift my head, open my eyes, move around in the chair and am wide awake.*

Many women have become very fond of this exercise and make it a daily ritual. Instructions that you give yourself in this deeply relaxed state have a way of becoming extremely effective. You can use this state to remind yourself that you will become even more relaxed the next time, and you will. You can remind yourself that you do not like fattening sweets and starches, and you will like them even less. You can make positive suggestions that can reduce worry and tension and improve self-confidence and assurance. But there is no time for that now—dinner is almost ready.

Squab for Dinner

The menu for dinner is a half of a roast squab on a platter with sliced tomato, sliced cucumber, lettuce leaves and radishes. Dessert is a half of grapefruit broiled for about three minutes. For the squab recipe see Appendix I.

Save the other half of the squab for tomorrow's lunch and the other half of the grapefruit for breakfast. Friday fish eaters may switch and have Saturday's dinner tonight, but then their lunches should also be switched.

Set the table for yourself even if you are alone. Arrange some flowers or light a candle for atmosphere. Make dinner a festive event and dine slowly as you enjoy each morsel. End the meal with tea and lemon or a hot demi-tasse. You may use artificial sweetener in either if you wish.

Doing Something Creative Can Give You a Lift

After the dinner dishes are out of the way turn on some classical music and devote one hour to some creative effort. If you do not paint, write, compose or sculpt, there is a gratifying sense of creative accomplishment in merely cleaning out a closet, straightening out a desk or arranging a few drawers. Bringing order out of chaos is therapeutic, just as therapeutic as creating a poem or an oil painting. Furthermore, it gives one a sense of a new start and that is the theme of this whole "pounds lost weekend."

You will find that the relaxation exercise which you enjoyed before dinner now enables you to do an impressive amount of work without feeling a bit tired. With no distractions and no pressure, work goes speedily and easily. One woman sent me a postcard during her weekend. She must have written it just at this point: "The relaxation exercises I did as I came to them. Found them delightful. Family had all left and I was alone in the house. When they came back it was 6:30. Where did the time go? After supper, family went to a show. I worked at my desk. Not a bit tired."

Stop at the end of one project. Do not let this new-found tranquillity and energy goad you into staying up until the wee hours. Set reasonable bounds and stay within them. For there is more work to be done before bedtime—on yourself.

A One-Hour Beauty Treatment

You are about ready to return to the kitchen. It's not to eat, but to prepare some beauty lotions. If you feel you must have something; put some water on to boil and have a social cup of tea or coffee with yourself. Here is the business at hand.

We want you to have softer, whiter hands. They are a feature of youth. This is how you can do it. Mix two ounces of oil of sweet almonds, two ounces of cocoa butter, and three ounces of lanolin. Heat in a double boiler, then allow to cool. Before you go to bed, you will spread the lotion on your hands and don the large-size cotton gloves which you bought earlier.

While this hand lotion is cooling, you may wish to use another one which is especially good for redness and roughness: dissolve a quarter of an ounce of alum into a beaten egg white. Massage into hands thoroughly. Wait until the lotion is stiff, then wash off.

While your night hand lotion is cooling, take your pick of any of the following facials. They vie with each other for popularity among movie stars and international beauties. Try one tonight, another tomorrow night: pure vegetable oil; chunks of watermelon massaged into the skin; any green leafy vegetable mixed in a blender and used as a face pack under hot towels; lanolin; fresh cream; almond oil mixed with mineral water; castor oil; mayonnaise.

Now you are ready for bed. Spread the now-cooled lotion you prepared on your hands, put your gloves on and turn out the lights. Do not think about any schedule for tomorrow. To do this will set your subconscious alarm clock to wake you early. Tomorrow will take care of itself. Sleep as late as you can. Pleasant dreams.

Saturday Morning Starts in the Cobra Position

Begin your day Saturday morning by stretching in bed. Keeping the legs straight and leading with the heel, lengthen first one leg, then the other, slowly several times. You will feel a gentle tug on your spine as it is stretched and relaxed. Now sit up and raise your arms so that they reach forward. Inhale in three sniffs wihout exhaling, then exhale and let your arms drop slowly. Repeat this breathing exercise three times.

You have just had what the yogi calls his first cup of coffee. You have awakened your body as yoga has advised for millenniums. Would you like to continue the body warmup?

Here is the next yoga step. It is called the "Cobra." It is graceful and easy to do. Lie face down on the floor or carpet. Place your hands on the floor alongside your chest as if you were about to do push-ups. You now slowly rear up, keeping your rear down. In other words, raise your head, neck, shoulders, chest, but keep your legs and hips immobile. You breathe in as you rear up, out, and come back down slowly. Do this three times.

There are a number of other yoga exercises that are stimulating to the body and rejuvenating to its muscles and tissues. Entire books have been written on the subject.[1] You have started the day ahead of the game. Perhaps when the weekend is over you may want to know more about yoga. But now it is time for breakfast.

How To Build Up Your Morale with a Different Breakfast

Have you ever shirred an egg? I know you have boiled, fried, and scrambled them, but eggs can be an exotic food. Ask the Chinese who have made an art out of preserving and pickling eggs. The oriental hundred-year-old egg is famous among gourmets. Follow the recipe for shirring eggs in Appendix I. Make your egg breakfast an adventure. Next time it may be an egg Benedict.

Set the breakfast table. Two spoons and a fork. One spoon for your half a grapefruit, the fork for your shirred egg, the second spoon to stir your hot coffee.

After breakfast, get dressed up. We are going into town to do some shopping. Do something you enjoy first thing in the morning and it sets the pace for your day. Even if it is only window-shopping, it is fun and exhilarating.

If you can, buy a dress, or a new hat or an accessory. A new dress can reflect the you that is being born, a new you who is chic and smart and eye-catching. Sweep into a fine dress shop like you owned the place. You will attract expert help and attention from the staff, which will sense your needs and be anxious to select the very dress for the new self you are projecting.

---

[1] Indra Devi.

Remember, you are still not ready for bright colors or shiny fabrics. Steer clear of splashy prints or checks, full or pleated skirts. Select from muted, solid colors, thin vertical stripes, and smooth fabrics.

Avoid wide or frilly hats, heavy jewelry, and button-type earrings. Simple hats with high crowns are for you. No, on belts; yes, on self-belts. Taller women can go for larger jewelry. Heavy legs call for darker stockings with seams.

Splurge a little. Make yourself feel good. It will last a lot longer than a banana split. Speaking of food, are you hungry? Stay away from that lunch counter. You are going home for lunch.

An Afternoon Adventure Helps Break an Unwanted Pattern

When you arrive home, try on that new dress. Look at yourself in the full-length mirror. Stand erect. Hold your tummy in. Shoulders back. Head up. Pleasant smile. You are getting there.

There's a half a squab awaiting you in the kitchen. Garnish it with watercress and some sliced tomatoes and lettuce. And how about a tall glass of iced tea or lemonade (using artificial sweetener, if you wish).

Take your time. Sit around over it. Play some music on the radio or hi-fi. Rest up. After all, shopping can be a strenuous exercise. What is more, you need your energy for the afternoon program that lies ahead.

I am going to ask you to do something this afternoon, preferably alone, that you have never done before. If you must take someone, all right, but I want you to feel your own zest and excitement. I want you to be uninhibited. "Oh, Mary, really!" That's a friend or relative talking. They do not expect you to do the unexpected. They want to hold you in the same mold that they see you in.

You are breaking out of that pattern. It is hard enough to break old habits without others offering resistance too. If you are lucky enough to have a husband, a boyfriend, relative or acquaintance who is out for new sights and new experiences also, lucky you; you have company for the afternoon.

What will it be? A walk up a nearby hill to see a view you have never seen? A trip to the zoo? A drive in the country to a museum, rummage sale or auction? A visit to a sauna or Turkish bath, a swim at the beach or pool?

Maybe you would like to go back to town and continue your shopping, this time for something you may never have bought before—like a wig, or wiglet.

Are you open to a suggestion? I would like to recommend a sauna, if there is one in your town or city. Here is why.

Let's Have a Sauna

Saunas have become a way of life in Finland. Finnish businessmen and politicians take their competitors and adversaries to the sauna. Hostility melts in the dry heat as the birch whisks swish, and stubborn moods open their pores to compromise. Rank and protocol, mask and pretense are shed in the dressing room with one's clothes. It is hard to maintain a pompous dignity in a birthday suit.

Women, blue-blood and commoners, react similarly to the treatment. There is something magical about the ritual. Steam rising from the hot stones. The dim light, wooden benches.

The public sauna bath house usually consists of a steam room, washing room and dressing room with separate quarters or times for men and women. The steam room is entirely of wood. Hot stones provide a constant source of heat. The sauna is usually maintained at a temperature of 175° Fahrenheit. Water thrown on the stones controls the humidity, a vent permits fresh air and temperature control. You sit on your towel, stimulate your skin with whisks of linden or birch, and watch the perspiration roll off and cleanse your pores.

The higher you sit, the hotter it is. It is best to start by sitting on the lowest bench or step. The heat steps up your metabolism. The increased flow of blood brings surging vigor to the body. In a few minutes you are ready to cool off in a shower before getting dressed.

What about your hair? Many women like to wash their hair while in the sauna. Steam has a way of making any coiffure look bedraggled, hence a shampoo in the sauna is an excellent idea. Many women rub oil into the scalp and cover their hair with a plastic hood before going in. Then the oil warms up and is absorbed, giving the hair a lovely lustre when it is washed. After shampooing, you can put your hair into curlers and sit in the steam room to let it dry. You can even use an electric dryer in most public saunas.

I want you to remember that I recommend the sauna as an exhilarating adventure, not as a means of slimming. Weight lost in the sauna is largely due to loss of body fluids, and a natural thirst soon makes up for it.

Have fun? Then it has accomplished its purpose. Adventure, new experience, is a hunger of the soul. Ignore it, and you are driven to food instead.

Saturday Night Is Devoted to Beauty

When you return from your adventure, you may be ready for a nap, especially if it included the great outdoors. Fresh air can make you sleepy. If you went to a sauna, you are ready for a nice long drink of cold water.

Rest up. Then prepare a late afternoon snack: Three soya crackers spread with a mixture of cream cheese and chopped watercress. Relax in front of the television set or with this book and enjoy the snack together with a glass of your dry sherry.

Now it is time for another relaxation exercise. Here is another relaxation technique that women find very effective. It involves mental images that have physical effect. Here is the way it goes:

How To Banish Ugly Tension Muscle by Muscle

Sit back quietly and comfortably and let your muscles go limp and heavy. Crease your forehead now, crease it tighter, now relax and let it smooth out. Now crease your brows and feel the tenseness. Let go, now close your eyes tightly, feel the tension. Now relax the eyes and let them remain closed gently and comfortably. Next clench your jaws, hold the teeth together as a vise, feel the tension throughout that area. Now relax your jaws and open the mouth a little. Now press your tongue against the roof of your mouth, feel the tension, then let go. Press your lips together tightly and now relax.

Now roll your head back as far as it will go and feel the pressure in the back of the neck. Roll your head first to the right, then to the left and feel the pressure change. Then bring the head forward and drop it to a position as close as possible to the chest. Now return your head to its normal position and feel the relaxation.

Now shrug your shoulders, pulling them forward and back, then around and around and now into a slumped position and feel the relaxation spread through your shoulders and upper back. Continue to keep the jaws and the neck and throat muscles easy and feel the tension leave and pure relaxation take over. Now breathe easily in and out and sense how relaxation increases as you exhale. Breathe in and fill your lungs, inhale deeply and hold your breath. Feel the tension. Now exhale and release the air automatically. Continue relaxing and breathe gently and easily and enjoy it. Continue to keep your body as relaxed as you can and fill your lungs again. Breathe in deeply and hold. Let go and feel the relief.

Now tighten your stomach muscles and make your abdomen hard. Feel the tightness—let the muscles relax and notice how they loosen. Again tighten and hold the stomach muscles and feel the tension. Release the stomach muscles entirely and continue to breathe normally and feel the gentle massaging action all over the body, particularly in the chest and stomach. Now pull your stomach in again and remain tense. Now release. Notice how after each time you breathe out you relax the stomach and the chest more and more. Try to let go of any contractions of the body, especially in the lower back. Arch up your back and make the lower back hollow if possible and then feel the pressure along the spine. Let go and feel the tension go. Arch the back again and try to keep the rest of the body as relaxed as possible while concentrating on the lower back. Relax once again, trying to release the tension more and more. Relax your lower back, your upper back, your stomach, your chest, your shoulders, your arms and face areas ever deeper, and more completely.

Now clench your right fist—clench it tighter and tighter and study the tension as you do so. Feel the tension in the right fist, hand and forearm and then relax. Let the fingers of your hand relax and see the difference in the way you feel. Now try to become more relaxed all over. Again clench the right fist and hold and feel the tension once more. Then let go and notice the difference once again. Clench the left fist, while the rest of your body relaxes, clench tighter and tighter, then relax and enjoy the contrast. Repeat once more, clench the left fist tight and tense. Now do the opposite of tension—relax and feel the difference. Continue clenching both fists tighter and tighter, forearms tense, study the feelings, let go, straighten out the fingers and feel the relaxation.

Now bend your elbows and tense your arms, tense them harder and harder and study the tension feelings. Straighten out the arms, let them relax and feel the difference again. Let the feeling develop. Once more tighten your arms. Now straighten the arms again so that you feel most tension in the muscles along the back of the arms, stretch the arms and feel the tension. Relax and get arms back into comfortable position. Let relaxation proceed so arms feel comfortable and heavy. Continue relaxing even further, even when the arms seem completely at ease.

Now flex your thighs. Flex your thighs by pressing down on your heels as hard as possible. Relax and note the difference. Straighten your knees and flex your thigh muscles again. Hold the tension, then relax hips and thighs and allow relaxation to proceed on its own. Press your feet and toes downward, away from your face, so that your calf muscles become tense. Concentrate on that tension. Relax feet and calves. Relax and keep relaxing for a while all over, including feet, ankles, calves, shins, knees, thighs, buttocks and hips. The lower part of your body will feel heavy as you relax still more. Now spread the relaxation to your stomach, waist and lower back. Let go more and more and feel cozy all over. Let the ease spread to your upper back, chest, shoulders and arms and right to the tips of your fingers. Make sure no tension has crept into your throat; relax your neck and your jaws and all the facial muscles. Keep relaxing your whole body like that for a while.

You may become twice as relaxed and calm as you are now by taking in a really deep breath and slowly exhaling.

Each time you exhale you become more and more relaxed and you can continue to relax for as long as you wish.

When you are ready to get up, simply count one to ten, each number will make you more and more awake and refreshed.

Are you ready for dinner? Tonight's menu is broiled fillet of flounder (six-ounce portion), broccoli spears with Hollandaise sauce (two tablespoons), and diet pudding (like D-Zerta). Recipes await you in Appendix I, but if your spirit of adventure has been whetted by this afternoon, improvise your own sauce for the broccoli, and draw on your own herb and spice resources to season the fish and bring out its fresh sea flavor to advantage.

Both the preparation and partaking of dinner is a joyous affair. It will be worthwhile if you time the preparation so that the fish, vegetables and sauce are at their peak simultaneously and you can enjoy them piping hot.

Beauty Secrets of Beautiful Women

This evening is beauty time. I am going to give you a number of beauty hints and let you decide which to adopt to transform yourself with a new youthful look. They have been collected from the beautiful women I know.

Let's start with your teeth. I mentioned in a previous chapter that crushed strawberries add new lustre to teeth. Use your fingers to massage the berries into your teeth instead of using a brush. If strawberries are not in season, a mixture of half salt and half bicarbonate of soda makes a fine tooth whitener. Here is one that is pretty far out, but on which I've had some good reports by the women who have used it. Take a slice of white bread that is now no longer for eating and burn it in your toaster or under the broiler. Burn it to a crisp. Then take the ashes, mix with salt and use as a tooth powder.

Next, your eyes. Take two tea bags, wet them and lie down; close your eyes and place them on your eyelids. You can do the same by dipping gauze in tea. Your eyelids are rested by the treatment, and this gives your eyes a younger look. To make your eyes brighter, use an eye cup and boiled water to wash them with a weak solution of boric acid. Now brush your eyelashes with cocoanut oil and notice how they thicken up and frame your eyes strikingly.

Wrinkles? Rub castor oil on your neck, chin, face or forehead.

How To Solve Persistent Hair Problems

Now to your hair. A variety of problems confront the woman in this area and they often turn her crowning glory into a crown of thorns. Hair can be dull, thin, oily, dry. It can be too straight or too curly. Here are a few problem-solvers that work and work fast:

For dandruff, mix a half cup of vinegar in a half cup of water. Wet hair with this solution. Dry lightly with a towel. No, beat an egg and massage it into the hair. Rinse thoroughly. Shampoo with a mixture prepared in the following way. Boil half a pound of pure castile soap in a quart of water until soap has the consistency of sour cream. Add one ounce of ethyl alcohol. Let cool. Shampoo and rinse.

Very dry hair can be helped in this way. Apply hot towel. Remove and apply a second hot towel. Remove and rub castor oil into scalp. Apply three more hot towels. Then shampoo out.

If hair is too oily, beat two raw eggs stiff. Brush into scalp with a toothbrush. Let dry, then brush out thoroughly. Another popular treatment, at least with my women, is to use a solution of powdered skim dry milk.

To thicken hair, use the same ingredient you did for eyelashes—rub cocoanut oil into scalp. It is a good daily habit to acquire.

For falling hair, mix the following solution: one pint of brandy, one ounce of white iodine, one teaspoon of salt and the juice of one lemon. Start by applying two hot towels, then massage the mixture into your scalp. Cover with hot towels for twenty minutes and shampoo out.

To bring out the highlights in your hair, there are three recipes for different shades of hair. For blonde hair, mix one cup of beer and the juice of two lemons. For brunette hair, vinegar in the rinse water. For white hair, use laundry bluing in rinse water, starting with a mild solution and working up till the desired white is there.

For general hair benefits, lemon juice is a light bleach, eggs give sheen and body, vinegar softens, and milk is a setting lotion that leaves no odor.

And so to bed.

Sunday, a Day To Think Young

I hope you have slept late and feel thoroughly rested. The pound or two you may have already lost this weekend should make you feel energetic, lighter on your feet, younger.

Before you dress, do your yoga exercise and get the benefit of its toning up. Extend the Cobra to the Swan. This is done simply by sitting back on your heels after you have pulled your head and shoulders back. Then move forward and let your arms lower you once more to a prone, face-down position. Repeat three times, breathing in as you rise, out as you descend, just as before.

Breakfast is delicious Welsh rarebit on a slice of whole wheat toast. See Appendix I for the recipe. Make fresh coffee. It does seem a waste to use percolator or drip for one person, but if you are alone, the extra flavor and aroma adds zest to the first meal. And remember, you can have a second cup if you wish.

Spend the morning relaxing over the Sunday papers or attending church. Think about the days that lie ahead. Do not dwell on the past, on all the gravy you ruined with skim milk, or all the time you have wasted beating your hips against door jambs to knock some inches off.

Think how you have fun as you lose weight in the weeks ahead and how your life will change as you become a younger and more beautiful woman.

The "big" meal of today is at lunch. We are having chopped sirloin steak smothered in sautéed onions. Broil four ounces of sirloin patty. Season well. Sauté one medium or large onion in a tablespoon of oil. Prepare six asparagus stalks the way you like them. For dessert have a fresh or canned plum.

Sunday afternoon you should socialize with family or friends. Do not discuss your "pounds lost weekend" with them but, of course, you can describe your adventure of yesterday, be it sauna or other.

Try to make it home early in the evening, because you have some beauty treatments before and after supper and before you retire.

Curl up in an armchair when you get home. Turn on the lamp next to you and, using the hand mirror from your vanity, examine your face closely. Notice how the lines of your mouth turn in a relaxed state. If there is a tendency for the edge of your mouth to turn down this is an indication of residual worry or tension. It can add years to your appearance. Practice smiling in the mirror, and trying to retain a residual smile when your face is relaxed.

How To Put Cosmetics to Work for You

Next, take our make-up and experiment. Have you ever tried a foundation cream? Select one the color of your skin or a bit darker. Apply it evenly over your face and throat using your fingers to blend it into your skin. You will find it removes harshness and creates a youthful look.

Next, scrutinize your eyebrows. Tweeze unruly hairs and those that make the brow line uneven. Tweeze a few to increase the distance between them. Use a sharp brow pencil to create a natural looking arch.

Eyelashes, when free of the falsies that are now so popular, can be accented with mascara used in moderation, or with the eyebrow pencil. Eye shadow can be applied sparingly to create more radiant contrasts.

Have you ever used a lipstick brush? You can create a more youthful look once you become adept at it. Tonight is the night to practice. Try adding fullness to your natural lip lines or filling them out differently than you have. Try a different shade. Seek to underdo rather than overdo.

If you approach the subject of make-up as if you were an artist, you can plan to fill your facial canvas to the best personal advantage, carefully choosing colors and shadings to blend harmoniously and to bring out your finest characteristics.

Dinner tonight is light. Make yourself a chef's salad. Let your imagination run wild. With your lettuce, include sliced cucumbers, celery, radishes, tomatoes. You may fill celery stalks with canned salmon or cottage cheese. Dessert is fresh or frozen strawberries (one-half cup). You may have your coffee or tea now or later.

After dinner plan to repeat the facial or hair treatment that you enjoyed the night before. Take a leisurely warm bath. Cleopatra used milk but you can get as much from water by using the high-protein treatments for hair and skin I have already described.

Give yourself a pedicure before retiring. Massage your feet with warm olive oil. If your problem is to keep feet dry, mix one ounce of powdered alum, one ounce of orris root, two ounces of oxide of zinc, and four ounces of talcum powder.

The time has come to close the blinds on your former self. As you turn off the lights and climb into bed at the end of the weekend, know that you are facing an entirely new tomorrow.

Review of Chapter Highlights

Mark next weekend on your calendar, or one in the very near future, as your "pounds lost" weekend. Try all the new ideas you have just read in this chapter in a weekend you will never forget. Shop ahead of time for what you will need during this special weekend. Plan on simple yet gourmet meals, accompanied by fine care. The agenda includes relaxation exercises, beauty treatments, and new adventures.

9

Psychology of Over-Eating—A Program
You Can Use To Lose Weight

Feelings, attitudes and emotions are at the base of every human problem. They start us on patterns of behavior, then leave us on them long after they have gone.

There is hardly a reader who can remember the pleasure as an infant of receiving a bottle of warm milk. It was comfort, security, love and nourishment all wrapped up in one delightful white package. But even though we cannot remember it consciously, we still reach out for nourishment when what we really seek is comfort, security and love.

No one is asking you to change that. The psychological law of "reverse effect" foretells that the harder you try, the more likely you are to fail.

The infant bottle quieted our aroused anxieties and hungers. Years later the morning toasted English, afternoon layer cake, and evening chocolates perform the same function. And still years later, even though the anxieties have long since disappeared, the habit— morning, afternoon and evening snacks—continues.

Hidden Causes of Obesity

A woman in her late thirties, pretty despite her size 42, told a group therapy session at a hospital obesity clinic at a large Eastern hospital that she had lost 35 pounds before dropping out of the last session. Then she backslid, regained 28 pounds, and here she was again.

The doctor in charge of the clinic suggested that she was angry with the group and that "hidden anger" is the cause of much over-eating. He described it as a passive, self-destructive kind of anger that finds outlet in the refrigerator.

This touched off a round of reactions from the women present. One woman broke into tears as she told how her husband sided with her fifteen-year-old daughter against her when she reprimanded her daughter over her poor grades. She immediately sought relief through eating. Another young woman, built on an operatic scale, complained of the kids being on her back all day and a backlog of work undone. She could not sleep that night and made several trips to the refrigerator.

Nagging husbands, rebellious children, husbands not home for dinner, and other frustrations were voiced by the women present at the clinic which sought to air these hidden causes, as a step toward emotional maturity. This group therapy, plus a low-carbohydrate diet, has made the clinic one of the most successful in the country.

This chapter will examine some of the ways emotions can affect eating habits. Then we will go into ways that proper habits can be restored. I promise you here and now it will be easy. No battles with will power. No pangs of conscience. No tears.

What Psychiatrists Know about Obesity

A recent psychiatric study in the United States involving twenty-five obese children disclosed that their families were characterized by discord and disharmony. Mothers were described in the study as being punitive, immature and domineering; fathers as ineffective, submissive, and undependable, or else as erratic and self-indulgent.

As you can well imagine, the children of these parents needed attention and love even more than most children, and probably received it less.

This does not mean that all of our overweight problems can be thrust on to the shoulders of our parents. The best of parents will reward a child with food and develop a conditioned reflex that lasts a lifetime: need for happiness and reward means a trip to the re-frigerator. The best of parents will give a restless, anxious child something to eat which they hope will act as a sedative. Another conditioned reflex is developed. Food equals peace of mind.

Case History of the Woman Who Gained Weight When Her Husband Was Ill

I hadn't seen Mrs. S. W. for seven years. At one time she had swung the balance of the scale to 175 pounds. After dieting with me she had reduced to 128 and had stayed there for many of the seven years.

Then, one day, she appeared in my office. I was shocked at the change in her. She looked unkempt and heavy again. She had in fact recovered 40 unwanted pounds.

She told me in a tearful interview of her husband's critical illness and how he now still was on the extreme danger list at a nearby hospital.

She was apologetic about her visit at a time like this, but remarked that despite his illness her husband was critical of her appearance and that she, too, felt the depression that always accompanied her obesity.

Her daily routine was shattered with long visits to the hospital and the hurried sandwiches obtained from the concessions.

We struggled back and forth with her weight until her husband was removed from the critical list and returned home to recover slowly. Mrs. S. W. then lost weight steadily.

How Structural Body Changes Begin

Psychiatrists find that beginning behavior patterns that are abnormal for one reason or another lead to structural body changes which tend to make the abnormality "normal." In other words, the body adjusts to overeating so that it is normal for that person to be fat. Try to reverse the process and you wonder why it is next to impossible. You think you have been trying to throw off a few excess pounds when you are actually trying to bend your body's processes from what has become normal and "right" for it to abnormal and "wrong" for it.

Of course, the body must be retrained. Longevity tables prove it is right to be slender. Men, with few exceptions, proclaim it is right for women to be slender. Your own natural intuition and instinct move you to be slender.

How do you retrain the body to accept slenderness as its norm. That will be the subject of the next chapter, but part of the success of that retraining depends on an understanding of the emotional causes behind overeating and how despite those causes, new eating habits are quickly and easily acquired.

A woman complained to me about a habit she had of biting her nails. She said she had been doing it ever since her childhood. As a small girl whenever she was nervous, worried or anxious she would bite her nails down to to the quick. Now she bit them anytime. Where someone else might doodle with a pencil, she bit her nails. It was obviously sheer habit. It fell away quickly and easily with reconditioning and retraining. It could have been midnight snacking or sweet toothing.

At the opposite end of the psychological spectrum is the compulsive eater. Now, many a woman has come into my office and confessed she was a compulsive eater. Ninety-nine out of a hundred were really not. Let me paint a picture of a compulsive eater for you, so you know once and for all, too, that the tragic shoe does not fit you.

The Compulsive Eater

Have you ever met anyone who could not stop eating? I do not mean the woman who takes one chocolate then another and another until she finishes the box. Or the chain potato chip muncher. Or even the whole-pie-at-one-sitting type. Believe it or not, these are not likely compulsive eaters. A real compulsive eater makes these people look like amateurs.

Case History of the Woman Who Lived—and Ate—Alone

A psychiatrist once referred to me a woman who weighed 350 pounds. The case history showed that the woman's weight problem began only two years ago, when she weighed 150 pounds. She had just been married. There was great disappointment when she found out she could not have a child. Within a year she had the marriage annulled. That was when she sought professional help, tipping the scales at 250 pounds.

She ate constantly, the psychiatrist reported. She lived alone—in the kitchen. When she went shopping she would be eating what she bought before she reached the checkout counter. When I checked her eating habits, I was amazed at the ingenuity she used to make sure she never stopped eating. I could not help the woman; there were very deep psychological forces at work. The food habit could not be dropped or changed while these forces were at work.

What were these forces? The woman could not fill her abdomen with child so she was substituting food. She ate to make her stomach big and she lived for that big stomach. The end of the story—at least as far as I know—came one afternoon when her land-lady called the psychiatrist to report that his now 300-pound patient was unconscious on the floor. When he arrived he found her in a heap of opened cans and miscellaneous groceries. She had tied pillows around her abdomen to make her stomach bigger. She was admitted to a mental hospital for treatment.

Are you a compulsive eater? I should say not. No forces compel you to eat after hunger has been satisfied or that full feeling attained. Your appetite can be turned off by food.

The Appestat and How It Is Controlled

The body mechanism that turns the appetite on and off is often referred to as the appestat. It is not a single gland or organ, but rather an interaction that produces the same kind of control for the body's demand for food as the thermostat does for the home's demand for heat.

The appestat is set basically by body needs, but it also responds to habit. The body can call for food through the appestat, but so can a tray of French pastries. It may be six hours since the last meal and your stomach empty, but it may also be only two hours since breakfast and time for your usual second breakfast. The appestat responds faithfully and the salivary glands reinforce its call.

The appestat controls the appetite. It tells you when to eat and when not to eat. Like the thermostat it can be set too high or too low.

Deep psychological forces can keep it on perpetually for those unfortunate compulsive eaters. Metabolic imbalances can cause the appestat to call for food when no food is needed, or to neglect to call for food when the stomach has been long empty. But usually the appestat's responses are normal.

How Emotions Can Affect the Appestat

To help you understand the tremendous effect that emotions can have on your eating habits, I must tell you of the rather stout mother who asked if she could bring her fourteen-year-old daughter to her second meeting with me. I told how I preferred to treat mother and daughter separately, but she was rather insistent, contending that her daughter would be terribly upset if she could not join her. Reluctantly I agreed.

The following week they arrived, the daughter barely a size less than her mother. Now, doctors often have a difficult time telling whether obesity in a child is inherited from an obese parent or whether it is what psychologists call identification. This is where a child imitates a parent. They like to copy the behavior of someone they love and respect.

There was no doubt in my mind, but I probed further. "Is this your only daughter?" "No," replied the mother. "My older daughter is at college." Then, perhaps sensing the purpose of my question, she added, "*She* has a beautiful figure."

By sharing her mother's life, and imitating it whenever she could, the young girl had found herself hungry when her mother was hungry, satisfied when she had eaten as much as her mother. Emotion had taken over her appestat. And her mother's craving for sweets, bread, cake and potatoes was mirrored every meal of the way.

Emotion can take over more than the appestat. Fear, guilt, jealousy, hate and other negative feelings can eat away at our stomach wall, causing ulcers, sap the strength of the heart muscles, harden our arteries and calcify our joints. There is not an organ in the body that cannot be damaged by the emotions. It is a wonder that the sensitive appestat is not thrown out of balance much more often than it is.

Case History of the Woman Who Was a Human Garbage Disposal

Mrs. J. P. was married at nineteen, just eleven years ago. She had five children, the eldest ten and the youngest age three. She entered my office hesitantly and was reluctant to stand on the scale. She guessed her weight at 192, but the balance showed 216.

She had weighed 132 pounds at the time of her marriage but her weight had steadily increased with the birth of each child. She now admitted to being at her top weight. She said, "The kids make me nervous; I always eat when I am upset."

I asked her to give me an idea of her everyday eating pattern. She didn't seem to know what I meant.

"Well, what time do you get up in the morning?"

"I'm up at 6:30."

"What is the first thing that you eat or drink?"

"Oh, I am never hungry in the morning."

"Nevertheless, what is the first thing that you eat?"

"I sometimes have a corn muffin or a bagel, but mostly I eat what the kids leave."

"What is the next time you eat?"

"Oh, I have something about 11, usually some coffee and a Danish. I told you I wasn't hungry in the morning."

"Do you have lunch?"

"I have to make lunch for the kids and I'll have whatever is around."

Mrs. J. P. was difficult to question. I have found it to be the best practice to ask a prospective patient to write down what they eat or drink four or five days prior to our first visit, otherwise I receive the kind of intangible responses I was getting.

"When is the next time you eat?" I plodded on.

"I don't usually eat any more until 4 o'clock, when I start making dinner and then I begin to pick."

"What does your usual dinner consist of?"

"Well, meat or something and some vegetables."

"Do you eat after dinner?"

"Yes, I pick all the time."

Mrs. J. P.'s problem was that she was without an eating system. She finished the kids' breakfasts and she ate whatever she made for her family for lunch and probably finished the leftovers too. Mrs. J. P. was one of the hundreds of female garbage disposals that I have met. She has probably spent hundreds of dollars on her various and sundry diet treatments and has saved pennies on food she should have thrown out.

We decided on a system. At 6:30 AM she would have a glass of orange juice and feed the kids their breakfast. Her breakfast would be at 8 AM, during which time she would give herself a half hour to eat and browse through the morning paper. Her morning meal would consist of some fresh fruit, one or two poached eggs, a slice of diet bread topped with her favorite low-calorie jelly.

She admitted to liking salads and 12:30 would be an ideal time for one. I suggested lettuce as a base, adding to it any shredded meat, fish, poultry or cheese that she happened to have around. Again her leftovers from her children's lunch were to be deposited in the garbage bag.

Four o'clock was to be her teatime. A cup of tea and no eating.

Breaking the picking habit while she was cooking dinner gave me the greatest problem. We decided she could pick while she made the family salad, since she could not go too far wrong on such ingredients.

Dinner was to be steak or chops, veal or lamb, poultry or fish, salads, vegetables and fruit.

It took me about a year to get Mrs. J. P. into the shape that she was in at nineteen. She has stopped being a human disposal and has become a svelte, beautiful woman.

An appestat can be functioning normally. Then something will happen in a woman's life. She can lose a boyfriend, have change of life, suffer financial setback. Next, her emotions can reprogram her appestat. Boredom in the guise of hunger can send her to the refrigerator. Insecurity, loneliness, the need for reward can make her hungry.

The appestat often reacts as if hunger actually existed. It sends out the call, loud and clear ("I think I'll treat myself to a piece of apple pie à la mode and a nice hot cup of coffee.")

If it seems farfetched to you for something as basically physiological as the appestat to be thrown off kilter by something as psychological as boredom, then you need to be reminded of present-day medical knowledge concerning psychosomatic medicine.

The Mind Can Do Strange Things to the Body

You need to be reminded that 25 percent of the heart attacks treated by physicians are brought on by escape, death wish and other deep-seated anxieties. You need to be reminded that attitudes and emotions are behind most cases of asthma, colitis, gall bladder trouble, gastrointestinal disorders, and other seeming organic problems. Every disease-causing germ gets the equivalent of an engraved invitation when the body's resistance is lowered by chronic worry and fear.

These diseases are all quite real, even though they are caused by the emotions and therefore designated as psychosomatic. The pain of a migraine headache is not imagined. It is due to the emotions, but this makes the pain no less intense. Many a blind person has been known to see, deaf to hear, paralyzed to move and dumb to speak when placed in a state of hypnosis. Such a state removes the mind-caused symptoms temporarily, and often they can be removed by the hypnotist permanently.

Yes, the mind can do strange things to the body and throwing the appestat out of balance is one of the least of these. Can the hypnotist correct this? Can anyone else? The hypnotist can reset the appestat quite easily and quickly. *So can you.* The next chapter will tell you how. However, it is based on symptom removal, rather than on cause removal. Although I have found symptom removal to be largely safe and permanent, there are instances where the removal of underlying causes is to be recommended. Let me explain.

Symptom Removal Versus Digging for Causes

Where psychosomatic conditions are impeding good health, the emotional causes behind those conditions can be treated or the conditions themselves can be treated. For instance, a woman complains of a fluttering heart. Examination by a specialist reveals no functional problems in the cardio-vascular system. However, she admits to hypertension over the fact that her husband has been seeing another woman. Question: Do you prescribe sedative drugs to quiet the flutter symptom, or do you counsel the woman, to prepare her to cope better with her marital problem?

There are those who say that to remove the heart flutter can lead to a more serious symptom. Like the woman who was made aware of the fact that her deteriorating vision was caused by family problems she did not want to see. The vision returned but she developed a brain tumor.

To satisfy the anti-symptom removal school, some psychotherapists and hypnologists resort to symptom substitution. They substitute a less harmful or less objectionable symptom for the one that is causing the problem. An involuntary muscular spasm in the shoulder, that made a social life impossible for one woman, was moved down to the little finger on her hand through hypnotic suggestion. There the spasm could remain as a physical outlet for some undetermined emotional cause without any further embarrassment or discomfort.

I have already used this method to help you. I have substituted eat-proteins for eat-sweets. The advantages are that there is no switch to another type of unwanted habit when the eating habit is suppressed, and there is less dependence on self-control.

However, there are many who feel symptom removal is safe for the preponderance of cases. They point to the medicines and drugs used by physicians, most of which is directed at alleviation of symptoms and totally ignores the underlying causes. I am inclined to favor this approach. I have yet to see any of my overeating women take on something else to excess when that symptom is removed. I am on relatively safe ground in the area of eating habits because if this is a necessary defense used by the personality, then it will fight my coaxing and not respond to the high-protein, high-enjoyment approach. Also, anyone seeking help, as my women are, are evidencing a desire to relinquish the symptom—in their case, overweight—once and for all.

It is more likely that the causes for adopting overeating as a defense have long since disappeared and the habit is ripe for ending. The infant's thumb succeeds the mother's breast, the pacifier succeeds the thumb. Then comes the lollipop. From there it can branch out to cigarettes or sweets or both. The search for oral satisfaction—begun as an essential need—winds up as vestigial habit or symptom ready to be dropped without aftermath.

Childhood Habits That Linger On and What To Do about Them

The need for oral satisfaction is not the only childhood behavior factor that can perpetuate its effects years later. How many parents give their youngsters a cookie or candy to keep them quiet and "out of their hair" for a few more minutes. The sweets become the habitual substitute for mother love.

Does the woman of thirty or forty who continues to hit the candy box as a daily treat to herself deserve to be called neurotic? I don't think so. I think she is doing what comes naturally to her, and what has been coming naturally to her for nearly thirty or forty years. She need not feel pangs of conscience and self-incrimination. She need only feel the need to change that habit, and follow the easy steps that will be spelled out in the next chapter to reset her appestat.

Some parents purposely build up a child's eating habits over and above the child's natural inclination. "Eat, grow big and healthy." The prodding reaches the subconscious habit forever. The child eats well, the big girl continues to grow bigger, and then as an overweight woman she wonders why.

What would happen, I wonder, if our childhood birthday parties, instead of the conventional cake, soda, candy and ice cream, featured barbecued steak or fish fillets. I am sure we would be less likely to consider those sweet carbohydrates as symbolic of joy and festivity. The steak and fish might take their place as the fun foods, right from the start.

Mother comes home from the bridge game. She asks the baby sitter, "Has Mary been a good girl?" "A very good girl," is the reply. Mother reaches into the sweet supply and out comes little Mary's carbohydrate reward. Years later, big Mary wonders why she hits the cake box when she's feeling low.

All of these childhood habits can be dropped by resetting the appestat, especially in the way I recommend, which reaches deep into those subconscious settings to make necessary adjustments. However, you may want to consider the treatment of some more recent habits acquired during adulthood.

Personality Problems That Put On Weight

Eating orgies are an adult failing. They can stem from a variety of adult problems. I love good food, imported wines and exotic desserts. But I don't go overboard. I find it quite rewarding to partake in modest amounts.

Occasionally something goes wrong. I eat too much. I know that my appestat has not been thrown off overnight. So I think back at the events of the past day or so. I find that very often my second- and third-portion meals come after a period of overwork and exhaustion. Another cause I have found is a rebuff by a non-cooperative client.

Feelings of hostility and frustration are common causes of over-eating, and of eating the wrong types of foods, namely the sweets and starches. Some people are starved for love and food becomes an easy substitute. Emotional hungers are many and edibles are the nearest thing at hand to feed them. Repressed marital unhappiness can lead men and women to seek extra-marital experience, but it is more likely to lead women to the refrigerator.

Often the crux of the problem is not that clear-cut. The overweight person cannot discern any crucial personality problems or emotional stresses even under the most rigid and objective self-evaluation. She is not unhappy, she is not tense, she is not frustrated, she is not worried. Yet she overeats.

I once asked such a woman who disclaimed being a worrier whether she worried about her climbing weight. "Of course," she replied. I pursued the point further and found that the reason she worried about the needle on the scale was that she knew the fatter she got, the less attractive she became, the greater was the risk to her health, and the less energetic and enthusiastic she became in her office job.

So she not only worried about her weight; there were other normal concerns for sex, health and job. These could not be entirely divorced from her basic emotional make-up and therefore from her eating behavior. It can be a vicious circle. Eating leads to concern, concern leads to eating.

There are clinics that treat obesity from the psychological approach. Their percentage of even temporary success is far under that of the milk farms and sweat boxes. Emotions are everywhere. Repress one, and there'll be another to take its place. Tailor your attitudes to tolerate others and life will deliver new experiences to cause different problems. And after you have successfully coped with all the emotions and attitudes, a Freud fan comes along and explains how all eating brings us erotic sexual pleasure and there is no sweeping that emotion under the behavioral rug.

Who knows? I personally prefer to stay on target. The target is the appetite. Let us see what we can do to set it straight.

Review of Chapter Highlights

How to take a long, frank, soul-searching look at yourself. How to put your finger on factors that might be throwing your appestat out of balance. Emotions can have a tremendous effect on the appetite, triggering hunger when actually the body has no need of more food. The original **cause** of overeating may have long since passed, but the **symptom** lingers on. How to recondition your attitudes and retrain your appestat.

10

How the Lazy Lady's Easy Diet
Reconditions You To Stay Thin

How do you change your over-
eating habits to stay thin without dieting? We know dieting is a
treadmill. It looks like it is taking us someplace, but in the end we
get nowhere. The answer to this question lies in the word "recondition."

At a London clinic recently, researchers removed the skull of
laboratory mice and studied what happened when they applied
various chemicals to portions of the exposed brain. One thing they
found was that they could make the mice continually hungry with
the use of some chemicals and cause loss of appetite with others.
Although these researchers had not discovered an appestat mechanism, they did conclude that such a mechanism existed and was
centered in the brain.

In another experiment with young chimpanzees, it was found that
by gradually increasing the amount of food given at each meal, the
appetite could be correspondingly increased. The more food given,
the more was needed. They were in fact causing an upward adjustment of the chimpanzee appestat by increasing the size of its meals.

If the appestat is partly controlled by how much we eat, then it
would seem to be a simple operation bootstrap to eat less, so we
could want less, and therefore continue to eat less.

That is the key, but it is not so simple as it sounds. As you well know, to eat less in the first place is an exercise in will power and we all know how the harder we try, the quicker we fail.

However, I have found some conditioning techniques that largely take the matter out of the hands of blind will power and place it more in the hands of our reason and intellect. For understanding of these techniques, I would like you to first explore with me the human appetite.

The Need to Fool the Appestat

When a woman comes into my office for the first consultation, I am interested in finding out what her capacity for food really is. Now, this is not easy to determine. Try asking yourself the question: How much fish do you eat in a portion—two, four, six or eight ounces? Or how much steak? In the absence of a scale on the dining-room table, the inclination is to pick a figure that *looks* right rather than *is* right.

I have had people tell me five or six ounces was their average portion of meat. No woman has ever confessed to eating a one-pound steak and yet most of them have, perhaps without knowing it. One pound is not a very big steak by restaurant standards, and at home it is so easy to reach for just one more small slice. (It is always a "small" slice.)

In order to get a standard to measure "small" by, I have a key question: I ask, "How much hamburger steak do you buy for your family when you go shopping?" I then ask how many hamburgers this makes, and how many she eats. It is a matter of simple arithmetic to divide the two or three pounds of meat by the number made and multiply by the number she eats to come out with a close approximation, at least with one food, of what "small" means. In the case of hamburgers I have seen "small" portions vary anywhere from three ounces to eight ounces.

I know I am going to have an easier time with the "small" eater at the eight-ounce hamburger level than I am with the "small" eater at the three-ounce portion level. In the former, the appestat is in need of adjustment. It is obviously set too high. It is quite a different matter to try to cool off a room where the thermostat is already turned low. Something else is out of whack. In other words, those who have been eating a lot will lose weight faster when quantity is cut.

Is that how you adjust the appestat—cut down on quantity? If we could manage to cut down easily, yes, that might be all there is to it.

But it is not usually easy to cut portions. The appestat resists adjustment in that manner. We have to fool the appestat. We have to perform some sleight-of-hand with food in order to make a little seem like a lot.

A Look Behind the Appetite Mystique

The appetite is a very complex and discriminating force. It hungers not only for quantity of food but texture, temperature, flavor and other contrasts. Even after the heaviest of meals we order a dessert. The appetite does not demand more food, but it does crave a change of pace.

Good cooks do not prepare meals where everything is of the same consistency. It would not be totally satisfying to the taste. Imagine chicken pot pie with dumplings—too much dough. Or rare roast beef with carrots and yams—too much red. Or Chinese egg roll with Chinese noodles and fried rice—too much fried in oil.

The appetite can be satisfied with far less quantity when we use textures, temperatures, and flavors wisely. Take steak. When you eat steak, you enjoy sinking your teeth into bite after bite. To stop at a half pound is to stop short of a full portion. A steak must be twelve ounces to a pound to be fully gratifying, and some people can do away with one and a half to two pounds without blinking an eye.

On the other hand, veal does not demand such oral activity. Veal cutlets are entirely satisfying in 6 to 8 ounce portions. Veal is richer, you say. That cannot be the answer, because a pound of steak is 1,600 calories, while a pound of veal is only 700 calories. In other words, a big eater who chooses steak consumes one pound or 1,600 calories, while a big eater who wants to fool his appestat, can choose veal, enjoy a large eight-ounce portion, and consume only 350 calories.

Compare 1,600 to 350 calories and you have a saving of 1,250 calories or, since 3,500 calories to a pound lost or gained, the equivalent of over one-third of a pound of human flesh lost. In other words, fool your appestat in some way like this every day, and you will affect your weight by more than two pounds a week.

Why 3,500 Calories Does Not Always Equal One Pound

Since I have mentioned that 3,500 calories of food are equivalent to one pound of womanly weight, I would like to detour for a moment to discuss this point. The 3,500-calorie figure is an approximation based on average conditions—average people, and an average diet. But people are quite different and their ways of eating are quite different. When you get right down to cases, very few people are average people and very few people eat precisely an average diet. So a 3,500-calorie reduction may mean more or less than a pound lost.

Some people digest less of their food than others. They excrete material that is less decomposed. Cut down 3,500 calories in the diet of such a person and it would not mean a full pound, since part of that 3,500 calories would have been excreted anyway.

The opposite is true for a person whose digestive process is at a higher level of efficiency. For her the 3,500-calorie drop in food intake makes a full 3,500-calorie internal difference, and the results on the scale would be that full pound and conceivably a shade more.

Some pretty dangerous reducing drugs and methods have been built around digestion. Mineral oil is a notorious example. Taken as a daily routine, mineral oil is an effective laxative, so effective it actually permits a greater percentage of food intake to be excreted. However, in doing so it exacts a health-wrecking toll. Absorptive tissues are coated and vital nutrients blocked from entry. The body is deprived of what it needs and malnutrition sets in despite a nutritionally rich diet.

One manufacturer claimed to have capsules that bloated in contact with stomach fluids and gave you that full feeling. Anybody care to guess what else it gave you? Your physician will advise you against the use of concoctions that purport to satisfy the hunger without adding food to the daily fare. Check with him before you take any reducing product.

The efficiency with which you digest food is but one factor that affects the 3,500 calorie figure. The rate of your metabolism is another. An excess of 3,500 calories over a period of time may not produce an excess of a pound in weight, if it is burned up by a highly stoked furnace. It would more likely mean that pound gained to a person with a banked furnace or lower metabolic rate.

This metabolic rate can be affected by the food itself. The protein food I have been recommending for health stimulates the metabolic rate, while the carbohydrate food I have been asking you to soft-pedal has a sluggish influence on the metabolic rate. Obviously 3,500 calories, cut in proteins is not going to have as much weight loss effect as 3,500 calories, cut in carbohydrates. The carbohydrate cut leaves you with a higher metabolic rate and a smaller waistline.

There must be other factors that affect this 3,500 calories-equal-one-pound ratio. For instance, I see every case history of weight loss go through periods of fast loss, slow show and plateaus of no loss. Every dieter reaches a time when poundage stubbornly refuses to yield. The pounds seem to hang on despite the lowered calorie intake, and if we lower it still more it seems to have no immediate effect. We need to make more radical cuts in carbohydrates or total intake in order to have the pounds begin to melt off again.

This seems to indicate that 3,500 calories equal one pound only at certain times for individuals, and I wonder, too, if 3,500 calories equal one pound for a small girl as well as a large woman.

Well, I did want you to be prepared for the arbitrary results of this 3,500 figure. It does not always follow that by cutting down 3,500 calories you will lose a pound and you should not be discouraged if you don't. One thing I guarantee you: You have a better chance of losing that pound by cutting down 3,500 calories of fats or carbohydrates. Now back to the job of satisfying our appetite while we adjust our appestat.

How To Make a Little Food Go a Long Way

I have told you how veal requires smaller portions than does steak, a high calorie-per-ounce meat. You can get away with smaller portions of steak by serving it sliced. Sliced tenderloin, or roast beef, or London broil seem to satisfy in servings of ten to twelve ounces rather than a pound. Chopped sirloin goes a long way, too, with eight to ten ounces a very adequate feminine portion.

In Europe, sizes of portions are generally smaller than in the United States. We are accustomed to larger portions in many types of food than most people would dream of serving in the other more economy-minded areas of the world. Training the appestat to be happy with less must overcome some of this conditioning we have that large portions are normal portions. If it looks any less than normal, we are ready to be hungry for more. Fool your own palate by using smaller quantities of spreads and eating them upside down. During World War II, there was a shortage of butter and fat in Germany. Germans discovered that they could make a little butter go a long way taste-wise by placing the sparsely buttered bread buttered side down in the mouth. The tongue thus came into contact with the butter and made it feel like much more than it really was.

Melon is a good case in point. A three-inch-wide wedge of honeydew, casaba, or cantaloupe is considered by most of us to be quite an adequate portion. But serve a three-inch-wide wedge of watermelon and listen to us holler. We are in the habit of huge, ear-to-ear chunks of this luscious red melon and anything less leaves us with a deprived feeling, despite the fact that it is just as nourishing in more modest portions as its smaller cousins.

You can fool your appetite and readjust your appestat simultaneously by resorting to the chop-and-slice technique in many foods. The watermelon portion can be thoroughly camouflaged by serving it in fruit cups, all cut into mouth-size pieces and depitted.

Almost any food you name lends itself to this technique. Ever hear of lambburgers or porkburgers? Lamb is delicious when ground and cooked like hamburgers. So is pork. And you eat far less than you would if it were sliced from a roast.

Another technique is to make a smaller portion take a longer time. We hear, so often that fat people bolt their food, hardly chewing it at all. I don't recommend that anybody try to change her chewing habits. The swallowing mechanism is about as involuntary and automatic as muscular reactions can get. One swallows without thinking when the food is ready to swallow.

I would prefer that you merely concentrate on enjoying the food you have in your mouth. In this fast-paced existence of ours, we often sit down to a meal and either converse, read the paper, or watch television simultaneously and are surprised to find the meal over. We have forgotten to taste what we were eating!

If you savour each mouthful, become more aware of it, you will eat more slowly and chalk up a much higher enjoyment factor for a much smaller meal.

How To Undermine Wrong Eating Habits

A woman complained to me that she had made protein-for-carbohydrate substitutions right down the line, but she just could not find anything to take the place of the danish she had with coffee sometimes twice a day. I think her problem is typical of that faced by 46 million overweight Americans who have developed a wrong eating habit and just cannot "kick" it.

The danish-and-coffee habit is quite prevalent. It got started, was compounded by repetition and then the pattern solidified. I explained this to my woman client who was failing in her valiant efforts to quit, and in the process beginning to feel quite guilty about it. "If you are neurotic, then so are 46 million others," I assured her. I explained how she was just manifesting a social condition based on a mode of living. It was a mode that placed time above food value. If something was available immediately and relatively pleasing to the taste, then it went well with the ten-minute coffee break.

If time has blugeoned you into an unwanted eating habit and if the pressure of time is holding you in that habit, then fight time, not the habit. Fold back time and take the pressure off. Vow to take three minutes or more to prepare for your coffee break, three minutes to utilize in the preparation of a suitable companion for that savory brew.

If you can prepare scrambled eggs in three minutes, and you enjoy scrambled eggs, you can displace danish from your coffee break. If you prefer a cheese omelet, and you can prepare a cheese omelet in four minutes, you will find it no sacrifice at all to forgo the danish. The sacrifice is in time.

What about those three minutes? Can you afford that much time each morning? I say you cannot afford not to spend those three minutes. When you consider that dumping a few hundred carbohydrate calories a day can mean two pounds a month or 24 pounds of unwanted bloat a year, three minutes a day is a small price to pay.

In fact, if it prevents your becoming overweight you are gaining time not losing it. Three minutes a day is only one day a year of waking time. But you can add years of waking time to your life span by preventing that 12 pounds of weight gain.

I proved to my danish-eating client that four minutes a day to fry some chopped meat to go with her coffee (this was her choice of substitute) would add four years or one and a half million more waking minutes to her life, according to insurance statistics.

If you care more about today than the future, let me put it this way: a few extra minutes to plan and prepare appetizing protein or low-calorie substitutes for carbohydrate or high-calorie habits can pay multifold dividends in new zest, stamina and vitality. When you feel and look years younger, you enjoy today more.

How To Put the Coffee Time Habit to Work for You

Take that time. Don't try instead to eliminate the coffee habit. You won't succeed, and it will only serve to discourage your efforts to get rid of sags and bulges. Cultivate the coffee habit and put it to work to slim and trim your figure. England used to have mandatory tea breaks at 10 AM and 4 PM; then they were discontinued. However, workers in many firms objected; they would sneak out to nearby lunch counters. The time they lost forced management to reinstate the breaks. The habit had been formed.

This stubbornness applies to all types of unwanted eating habits. As a result, you have to let the habit stand but change the ingredients. Don't wrestle with the quantity. Instead, shift to the protein side of the food spectrum and shift to lower-calorie type foods.

I know one office girl on the plump side who was able to break the association between coffee and cake by switching to black coffee. "I concentrated on the flavor of the coffee," she said. "By drinking it without cream or sugar I was able to smell the aroma better and savour the flavor of the bean. It took my mind off the missing English muffin."

If even strong black coffee remains as a "cake-triggering" mechanism for you, you may want to try dumping the coffee in favor of some other types of midmeal snack, such as yogurt or fruit. Or, a different type of beverage—like tea, or manufactured beverages.

Most people favor the sandwich for the lunch break. *Two slices of bread are too carbohydrate-high.* One slice of bread is twice as good for you as two. Take off the top slice and fold over the bottom. "I do better than that," said twenty-five-year-old social studies teacher. "I have the cafeteria manager in my school trained to give me the contents of the sandwich on a plate with a sprig of lettuce and parsley." Great. Any restaurant will do the same for you. A hamburger *without* the bun. (Have a double, if you like. You are still ahead in the "thinning" game.) Salmon salad on white, tuna on rye—all make appetizing salad plates, but sans bread.

Case History of the Family of Five That Weighed 1,150 Pounds and Lost 400

Once in a while I have a whole family to deal with. This was one of those times. The husband was a 350-pound architect; the wife a 200-pounder. Two daughters, aged seventeen and nineteen, weighed almost 400 pounds between them, and a son of fifteen tipped the scales at 158 pounds. This type of case is usually easier than that of an individual attempting to diet while everyone else is knee-deep in seven-layer chocolate cake.

There was a complication. The children, although terribly obese, were very picky eaters. The son did not eat vegetables, fruit, or fish of any kind. The daughters' habits were to prefer sandwiches over any meal, while the parents loved spaghetti or pastas in any form.

Eventually, after a number of false starts, menus were arranged to fit the family. They were based upon a seven-day plan. Each day there was some small compromise from some member of the family. The mother, who was the most difficult, responded well. Within six months the family lost an accumulated total of almost 400 pounds.

The Importance of Planning

"I went out for dinner last night and blew everything," a mother of three confessed to me. "What happened?" I asked. "I had every good intention of ordering veal scallopini," she explained, "but when I read the flowery descriptions on the menu and saw the steaming lasagne go by, I succumbed to temptation."

Where did she go wrong? Her intent was right, but I say it was not strongly backed up with planning. She should have spent a little time on that veal scallopini. She should have recalled how delicious it was at that restaurant the last time she had it. She should have reviewed how low the calorie or unit count compared to other choices. She should have visualized herself walking into the restaurant, smelling the Italian spices and aromas, seeing the spaghetti and the pasta, and ordering the veal scallopini.

Planning means more than making a decision. It also means planning how to implement that decision, how to proceed to carry out your decision despite all obstacles.

These obstacles usually take the form of temptation. There may be additional effort involved or additional time, but temptation is the main pitfall. A mother whose 145 pounds did not sit too well on her 5-foot frame was faced with a yen for apple pie. She could plan a substitute for herself easy enough—a gelatin-type pudding—but her family insisted on that pie several nights a week. She was able to serve them the pie for dinner while she enjoyed her special pudding, but then, she said, she could not resist going to the refrigerator later for a slice. "Just knowing it was there," she said, "turned me into putty." We beat the problem with one more step in the planning. Whenever she planned pie for the family, she selected one neighbor who was going to get an unexpected after-dinner visit from a good-hearted woman who had some leftover apple pie. It worked weight control for the mother, and her neighbors would have voted for her for President.

The obstacles of time and energy need this extra planning, too. Plan what time you will have to start dinner in order to complete the preparation of the fondue you are having tonight instead of pizza. Go over the ingredients you need. Shop ahead of time to make sure everything is on hand.

When you do this planning, recognize what you are accomplishing. Understand that the mental images are actually reinforcing your decision by reprogramming your subconscious motivator.

Soon you will find you are completely ignoring old reactions to certain foods. You are breaking former compulsions. You recognize that you are controlling your own behavior. You are no longer a slave to an uncontrollable appestat. You are controlling that appestat. You begin to realize that you have the responsibility over yourself. You can no longer blame glands, nerves, metabolism. You cannot call yourself neurotic or compulsive and go about your old eating habits blameless in your own eyes. You are the captain of your weight, and you have set your course, and nothing, but nothing, can interefere with your complete control of your weight.

How To Recondition Yourself Against "Problem Foods"

Finally, I want to give you a technique to knock out those few foods that have such a hold on you that all of the before-mentioned planning is not enough to cope with them. The method I am going to give you now is the knockout punch for and of those weight-wreckers that persist in upsetting the appestat and sliding pounds back on you.

Follow these instructions step by step, and you will be rid of these villains in a few days. First, I want you to list the foods you know to be high in calories or carbohydrates, or both, which survive despite all your menu-planning to the contrary. Put the toughest villain last, the easiest first on the list. Conquer number one before you start on number two and proceed right to the next until you have dealt that knockout blow to every single item on the list, working up to the toughest last.

Ready to start? Let's say the first on your list is ice cream. You can take or leave it, but you usually take it, maybe two or three times a week. The action I am about to describe to you, you can accomplish just as soon as you read it now, by simply putting the book down and following simple instructions:

See yourself being offered ice cream and refusing it. See yourself passing it up at a restaurant, soda fountain, your own kitchen. Know beyond a shadow of a doubt that you can refuse it. Play the scene over a few times in your mind's eye. See that there is no effort, no will power. You refuse ice cream effortlessly, willingly, unfailingly. Now try it.

Why does this work? It works because that is how we motivate most of our actions initially. Then habit takes over. You imagined putting your spoon into ice cream and eating it so many times that it became a habit.

Does it work on the first try? Yes, but you may have to reinforce it from time to time. When you go to the next item, you will include ice cream again. So your second mental exercise will not only get rid of unwanted item number two but it will reinforce your first mental exercise.

Another way to reinforce those mental exercises to rid yourself of hard-to-shake foods is to relax thoroughly first. Use the relaxation exercises I provided for the "pounds lost weekend" in Chapter 8. Relaxation permits new mental images to sink deeper into the subconscious where they replace the old.

If bread is item number two, do not start until you have had a chance to see how well your exercises have worked on item number one—ice cream. You have listed ice cream first because it is easiest. Eliminating bread will be harder. But when you see success take place, that success reinforces your belief and expectation. Confidence builds up. Your skill in relaxing and visualizing improves. You find ways of including sustitutions in your imaging ("I see myself eating salad instead of potatoes").

If your list is long, it is hard to visualize ten or twelve foods one after another. Lump them together after a while with some term like "junk." Ice cream, bread, potatoes, etc., are visualized as a glob of fattening "junk." You see yourself refusing even to go near this "junk."

Do you know that a jelly doughnut can actually put an eighth of a pound on your buttocks? Think of it. That "junk" is not just "junk";

it can become overnight that ugly loose fat and flab, the sag, bulge or spread. Understand just how "junk" is digested, separated, transformed and carried by the blood to ribs, hips, etc.

How To Use the Mirror Figure

Stand in front of a full-length mirror. Scrutinize your figure carefully. Note where the unwanted ounces and pounds are. Now, looking at these bulges, associate them with the food items on your unwanted list, "the junk."

Do this exercise to extremes and it will be amazingly successful. I remember how one woman described her mirror extremes. She said she stood in front of the mirror in the nude for five minutes. She measured her hips and thighs. She poked and slapped herself and watched the flesh shake. "I had avoided looking at myself in the mirror this way before. Now I faced up to my fat. I reminded myself that my protruding stomach was pure spaghetti, my layers of waist pure potatoes." It worked for her. The image stuck and the sight of potatoes on someone else's plate touched off revulsion where once they spelled temptation!

I hope I have given you an insight into what makes your appetite tick. It has been ticking away all these years and all these pounds. Now you can control that tick. You can adjust your appestat, control temptation, and knock out fattening foods. All without will power, diet, and frustration. The world of radiant beauty, brimming health, and successful living awaits your mental bidding.

Review of Chapter Highlights

You can retrain your appestat by eating small portions that look big. How to include on your menu effective appetite-fooling tricks. Taste, texture, temperature and flavor of foods can work against quantity of food desired. A high-protein diet generally gives you a higher metabolic rate and therefore you burn up more calories in losing weight. Visual exercise on page 130 that reconditions you against craving problem foods.

11

Low-Calorie Cookery and Satisfying
Snacks for Weight Control

"If I didn't eat between meals, I'd never be able to stick to that diet I'm on." It is often said in jest, but there is a great deal of truth lurking in the humor.

A successful weight-watcher is not necessarily the person who fastidiously avoids between-meal snacks. You can well be the person who knows just as well what to eat for weight control between meals, as during meals.

Dieting is easy if it permits you to enjoy eating what you like and when you like. It may not get the weight off you so fast as many popular crash programs, but the weight will stay off. You have no disciplined regimen to end and the fun way of eating to return to. You are already on the fun way, with great dividends in health and beauty.

The axiom of three square meals a day has no physiological basis. It is a social custom in the civilized world, but no more. Journey into the bush country, and you soon find breakfast, lunch and dinner times give way to meals when you are hungry and the food is available.

I propose that you eat when you are hungry and that you make sure that food best for you is available. The only hitch is I don't recognize carbohydrates as food. At least they are not food in the sense that proteins, fats, minerals and vitamins are food. Carbohydrates in their purest sweet and starchy form do nothing to nourish your body adequately, build your health or enhance your beauty. Quite the contrary. Candy, cake, pie and cookies can sap your body's strength, undermine health, and make you ultimately fat and unattractive.

I say eat as many as eight meals a day if you wish. But eat and snack the low-carbohydrate, low-calorie, high-nourishment way.

Ways To Cut Carbohydrates in Cooking

It's peculiar how flesh and fat of animals turns more slowly into flesh and fat of humans than does the carbohydrate burned for energy. But science confirms that protein tends to step up metabolism, carbohydrate to slow it down. Furthermore, the very act of digesting proteins requires from six to eight times more internal energy per ounce of food consumed than does the digesting of carbohydrates.

The poets and writers of the past millennium appear to have associated fat with anything except carbohydrates. "Fat as a whale" was Chaucer's simile, and a whale has only a trace of carbohydrate. "Fat as butter" said Shakespeare, "Fat as a barndoor fowl," Congreve; and "Fat as seals," Hallock—all devoid of fatty carbohydrate.

"I was counting my day's carbohydrate calories last evening and it suddenly struck me I had forgotten to count the batter on my fried chicken. It ruined my total. Must I give up fried chicken?" The question came from a blonde housewife who had lost two pounds a week for three weeks and was anxious not to break her weight-losing stride. To me the answer was obvious. I have been frying chicken for years—without batter or crumbs—and I would not dream of giving it up.

I love to cook. I get a great deal of enjoyment revising recipes to lower their calorie count and to squeeze the carbohydrates out of them. I have on hand hundreds of recipes that have been developed for high-enjoyment and low-calorie value. Most of them started in my clients' kitchen files and then went through the Petrie process of adding necessary nutrition value and subtracting unnecessary fattening value.

In Appendix I you will find a selection of these recipes. I have taken out sugar and starch and added everything from aroma to zest. The total calories per serving and the total carbohydrate calories per serving are listed for each, so that you can evaluate them for your own program.

I can sum up the chief shortcuts to low-carbohydrate cooking as follows: Omit sugar, omit flour. Now, I sometimes substitute an artificial sweetening for sugar, and I sometimes substitute wheat germ for bread crumbs and batter. But, by and large, even these substitutes can be bypassed with some creative spices and sauces.

Feasts You Can Enjoy from Faraway Lands

I get a great deal of my food inspiration from exotic foreign lands. With the exception of rice and pastas, I find most foreign cuisine contains far less carbohydrate-heavy ingredients than American. So I avoid the rice dishes, and doughy recipes. When I come to a Chinese recipe that calls for cornstarch, I omit that ingredient. It may not thicken up the dish but it does not thicken me either! Sometimes I substitute arrowroot. It is lower in calorie value and higher in nutritional value.

"What is this? It's delicious!" I seldom give away my secrets. I let them analyze it for themselves. Sometimes it takes away the glamour to put it into words. Like my escargots au beurre. Some people don't like snails. Or my sashimi. Now how in the world can somebody be squeamish about raw fish? It's only fresh tuna or sea bass dipped into a tangy shoyu sauce with ginger bits. Not a calorie or carbohydrate in a carload.

Appendix I is just a small start for you. Open up some of the cookbooks you already have. Buy some of the new crop that is published every year. Open up your horizons to include food of many lands. There is every reason why, as calories drop, weight drops, but enjoyment can zoom.

Why does cheese taste so good when it comes from Europe? Wisconsin, Vermont and other states have splendid cheese. I have tasted cheese as it formed in vats in Wisconsin dairylands and seen giant cheddar wheels aging in the coolness of Vermont caves. This is great cheese. I am not talking about the pasteurized, colored, processed or artificially flavored. I agree that does not equal the imported varieties. But we do have fresh whole milk domestic cheeses, some that are natural country aged, some that are smoked golden over hickory log fires. Unsurpassed. Yet we find the connoisseurs ordering French roquefort, Danish blue, and Swiss gruyère. I believe the answer lies in the degree of craftsmanship. European cheesemaking has been perfected over the centuries and the skills passed on from father to son.

Perhaps that is the reason why so many countries have developed reputations for good eating. Their sauces, seasoning and other culinary secrets have been developed over many, many years. Ours is a relatively new country. We do not have much more than the frankfurter and the hamburger to brag about and even these are named after German cities.

Knowing of my interest in foreign cuisine, a mother of a sixth-grade boy invited me up to a celebration of United Nations Day in the school. She and the other mothers each brought authentic dishes to an international lunch. I saw teriyaki from Japan, golatopouku from Greece, strufoli from Italy and a score of tantalizing delicacies. Neither she nor her husband had other than American parents and grandparents, so she represented the United States with Yankee Doodle apple pie.

We cook chicken usually in one of three ways—broiled, roasted or fried. We sometimes serve it in a pie or fricasseed. But that's about it. The French serve it in a pot au feu, the Polynesians baked with pineapple, the Congolese sautéed in palm oil, the Persians boiled, then deboned in rose water. Chicken is an international food and although one can be bored eating it the same way all the time, there is no law preventing you from crossing international boundaries at the stove and making chicken a new travel adventure each time.

I do not have to show off my skills with the skillet. There are international recipes in daily newspapers, magazines and cookbooks. But I do want to encourage you to experiment and break out of the usual kitchen routine. You can heighten your taste experiences with new dishes and therefore be satisfied more with what you eat. I have already explained how heightened satisfaction serves to cut down servings and keep you on a slenderizing fare.

Health Hints in Cooking from Abroad

In previous chapters I have reviewed the important minerals and vitamins, what they do for the body, and in what foods they are most commonly found. Health and food are closely related and, needless to say, the selection, combination and preparation of foods are equally closely related to health. Here, too, skill comes with experience and there is much we can learn from other older countries of the world.

Sometimes it is less a question of knowledge though than it is of ignoring knowledge for the purpose of economy and expediency. Take fruit. Sun-ripened fruit is by far more nutritious and easily digested than the brand most of us eat that ripens aboard ship, plane or train. Yet, unless you live by an orchard, the chance to savour a naturally ripened pear or peach or plum or banana has not even a once-a-year likelihood of happening. In Europe, Asia and Africa, fruit is brought to nearby markets much more often than it is shipped to far away cities. The local village market is replete with fruit of the season. We who live in the city can do little about this, except to remember to stop at our own local farm stands when in the country and look to treat ourselves to the nutritional power of sun-ripened fresh produce. The practice of growing one's own herbs, parsley, and vegetables is spreading in our suburbia. Also more and more Americans are discovering dandelion greens, wild onions and the asparagus-like tender shoots of poke weed.

The French eat much greener salads than we do. Our white iceberg lettuce may keep longer in transit and on the shelves, but the French realize that endive, romaine and escarole types of green lettuce taste better and are richer in nutrients.

The French long ago discovered the value of brewer's yeast. Today French people make it a way of life. It is available in tablets or powdered form almost everywhere that food is sold. Also, sweet desserts never did get a foothold in Paris. Cheese and a piece of fruit is still on the best-seller list.

Picking an example on the other side of the world, the Chinese the Japanese look to the sea for their treasure trove of nutrition. Fish in every form and even seaweed are revered for their taste and health value. Japanese enjoy many varieties of sea herbs, sea kelp and sea lettuce, all rich in minerals and nutrients, especially iodine and that newly discovered vitamin K.

Orientals undercook their meat, fish and vegetables to preserve the natural flavor and nutritional values. Chinese use sesame or soy oil and a heavy hot pan. The quick cooking leaves the vegetables tasting crisp and fresh, especially compared to the overcooked variety served up at the average American home.

In the Middle East, seeds are the secret to health and longevity. Sesame, sunflower and pumpkin are chewed the way we chew gum. Only they are true foods that carry within them the germ of life.

Russians munch on sunflower seeds, instead of popcorn, while attending the cinema. Sunflower seeds have high calcium, iron and phosphorus content, as well as B vitamins and niacin. The hulled seeds can be ground into a meal and used in meat loaves. In India, sesame sweets are obtainable in many tempting delights. Here, too, sprouts of the living mung beans, cultivated in two or three days between wet blotters, are eaten for their germ of life potency.

I would sum up the health lessons to be learned outside of our country as:

1. More sun-ripening of fruits and vegetables.
2. Greater use of fish and sea plants.
3. Greater appreciation of yeasts and yogurts.
4. Smaller amounts of water or oil used in cooking.
5. Attention to the vital life properties of seeds, wheat germ and sprouts.
6. Popularity of such higher protein grains as millet and buckwheat groats.
7. Greater variety of leafy vegetables in soups and other dishes.
8. Wider use of raw foods and less cooked-through dishes.
9. Smaller portions and fewer meats.
10. Greater appreciation of food preparation as a craft.

Other countries have much to learn from us, too. But, by using the best of the world's tried and true, we can become more vibrantly alive, more creative and productive, and more energetic and youthful.

The Truth about Organic Foods

Much has been said, written and argued about natural and organically grown foods. Are they more nutritious? Is it more healthful to eat foods that are in the form nature has produced them, or can man's manufacturing skills improve them?

The controversy develops because people can be burning with health on both. The natural food enthusiasts talk about the dire peril of devitalized and overprocessed foods, while most of the very people who eat them are in fine health. The processors ridicule the claims of the natural food enthusiasts, while the latter display their fine health.

I am not interested in taking sides. I am interested in leading women to the most nutritious and delicious foods for the least amount of calories, especially carbohydrate calories. Your prime interest in the subject should be identical.

There are certain facts that are not controversial. There is no doubt that the processing of rice, sugar, and wheat removes material that is laden with nutrients. Whole-grain flours are more vitamin- and mineral-rich than refined flour. There is no doubt that baking soda and baking powder are less healthful as leaveners than yeast, with its valuable vitamins, or egg white, with its valuable protein. There is no doubt that fruits and vegetables grown in rich soil are more healthful than those grown in depleted soil.

Given the choice, which would you prefer: fresh fruits and vegetables just picked, or packaged fruits and vegetables that have been on the shelves for months and maybe years? Packaging techniques are better today than they have ever been. Foods are being preserved more efficiently and longer. But regardless of the excellent packaging, the only items I feel improve with age are meat and cheese to a point, and liquor. Other foods may not deteriorate drastically but they are certainly no more vital at the end of their storage period than they were at the beginning.

Denatured wheat and polished rice have been separated from the principle of growth inherent in the germ of life. They have more calories per nutrient. If you seek more nutrients per calorie, I recommend whole wheat, wheat germ, and brown rice. They have more tissue- and bone-building items.

Converted and processed foods take less time to cook. But are we trading those few minutes a day for bloatedness and flabbiness? Too much of the nutrients of food are lost between the time they are in contact with the sun and rain and contact with the human mouth. We need to retain these nutrients wherever possible. If we cannot control the planting, the fertilizing, the growing, at least we should try to get to the fresh foods as rapidly as possible and prepare them in their most complete and original form.

This preparation can be, in itself, the demise of much of the nutritional value. If a vegetable rich in water-soluble vitamins and minerals is soaked overnight, the water that goes down the drain carries with it most of those blessings. If a vegetable or fruit, endowed with minerals in its skin, is peeled, the garbage can see the benefits.

A recipe tells us to let the pot simmer all day, but it does not tell us the nutritive value of a food is decreased by long cooking.

Another recipe says to beat with an eggbeater until foamy, but it does not tell us that contact with air destroys the vitamins.

Build your own health and vitality by taking a greater interest in the vitality of the food you eat. You will reflect that interest by a new radiance beyond anything you have experienced before. Family and friends will confirm this with compliments.

The theory behind organic farming is this: A depleted soil can produce only depleted food. Try to pep up this soil with chemicals and chemicals, not nutrients, appear in the food. On the other hand, renew this soil by putting plant and animal fertilizers back into it, and the soil begins to teem with bacteria and microscopic life that produce natural minerals and vitamins which then appear in the food. As I said before, I am not going to take sides. I leave the decision to you.

Low-Calorie Snacking

A twenty-four-year-old secretary with her eye on a modeling career showed me in jest a diet she said she was on. It contained such items as one doughnut hole, a glass of dehydrated water, and three ounces of prune juice (gargle only). We enjoyed a good laugh over such "low-calorie" items as scraped crumbs from burned toast, boiled out stains of a tablecloth, and aroma of empty custard pie plate.

Seriously, some diets are inhuman. They have built-in failure. Nobody but nobody could maintain her spirits much less her body on the bouillon-cube lunches and carrot-stick dinners that I have seen women on. Can you blame them for snacking in between?

You will snack less on a mildly reducing, low-carbohydrate, high-protein diet. You will not feel pangs of hunger driving you to the refrigerator, but if you do wish to snack, you will not feel pangs of conscience for doing so, either.

"I could hardly believe that I am on a diet at all," writes a woman from Dallas who followed the low-carbohydrate way in one of my previous books. "Before I started with this I seemed to be eating all day long without really tasting my food at all."

Tasting is vital to the act of eating. If you do not enjoy the taste of a snack, it will not count. If you do enjoy it, you will be happy until meal time. Therefore an enjoyable snack, even with a few calories, taken once, is more slimming than, say, a salty potato chip or pretzel taken again and again and again.

Here are some examples of what I mean. Underscore the ones that appeal to your taste.

Mushrooms have almost no calorie value. An extremely large one is only one calorie. Now, if you were to mince some low-calorie clams, mix them with pulverized matzos instead of bread crumbs, sprinkle with parmesan cheese, brush with a half teaspoon of margarine, you can broil yourself a tray of gourmet snacking that will be like a meal in pleasurable eating. Put the rest away in the refrigerator for tomorrow.

In Thailand, there's a dish called yumpatu. All it really is is tuna fish mixed with lemon juice, finely chopped celery and green onions, and served chilled on lettuce leaves. All I am eliminating from this snack are the peanuts that the Thais sprinkle on the top. Even without the peanuts, yumpatu is a satisfying snack and a conversation piece at a cocktail party.

Case History of the Star Who Lost Weight At Parties

Although many of these case histories are about grossly obese persons, in the main, the majority of women that I see are perhaps 7 to 20 pounds overweight. Such a case was that of Miss B. E. I have even disguised the initials, for the lady is famous in the world of entertainment. She had a secretary to arrange all of her dinner and cocktail dates. I asked her to make a list of what she ate at these parties for a period of one week. The case was an easy one—the exchange of straight liquor for whiskey sours, the selections of shrimp, crabmeat, meat balls, cocktail frankfurters and other high protein foods for the canapés and potato puffs. That is all I had to do. It made all the difference between an unhappy star and a flat-tummied one!

The Fascinating Hunt for New Low-Calorie Ingredients

My feminine gourmets are this very minute planning new tasteful combinations of low-calorie ingredients. Like hobbyists, they collect these ingredients with skill and interest, exchanging them for unwanted high-calorie, high-carbohydrate ingredients.

Two very basic exchanges are using artificial sweetener instead of sugar, and soya bean flour instead of regular flour. Flour is normally 358 calories for four ounces, while soya bean flour is 290 calories. But what is more, the different density of these flours saves you added calories—it takes about four and a half ounces of regular flour to make a cup, but only four ounces of soya bean flour. This means that a cup of regular flour is 400 calories, compared with 290 for soya.

Supermarkets now carry butter and margarine in brands with only half the normal calories. Using these as shortening, artificial sweetener in place of sugar and the soya flour, you can come up with homemade crackers that are not fattening, to use with spreads.

Half-the-calorie-count cheeses are now available. Furthermore, the calorie value of any cheese can be cut in half if the cheese is heated and used as a spread. The calorie cut occurs in this manner because only half of the normal quantity is necessary. Shelves are filled with new diet spreads. There are low-calorie jellies and jams.

If you do not like the taste of diet canned fruit, you can reduce the calories of regular canned fruit considerably by washing. Pour off the syrup then fill can with tap water and pour off. I have found that this does not affect the taste.

The sodium content of canned fish or meat can be reduced by washing five minutes under cold water. This is extremely important to dieters with water-retention problems, as your physician will confirm.

Sandwiches made of thin white diet bread (by cutting the slice in half horizontally) only adds 40 calories for one sandwich. Two slices of ordinary bread would add 140 calories for one sandwich. Incidentally a housewife can roll a slice of diet bread to about twice its size, spread with a filler such as tuna, then roll into a cylinder and cut in slices for party treats.

Most cakes can be made with low-calorie flour, fresh fruit and half-calorie shortening and in this manner their calorie content is reduced.

For example: A slice of jelly roll 3″ in diameter is normally 350 calories; however using these ingredients and low calorie jellies it can be produced for 110 calories.

More Kitchen Tips, for Slimming Your Figure

Earlier, I told you of how replacing beef by veal can cut calories. This exchange in hamburgers or meat loaf can mean a savings of 50 percent or more in calories. Meat mixtures are popular in swank diet resorts in England. Baked meat loaves and hamburgers are made by combining ground chicken and ground veal with beef, to lower the calorie count. Combinations can be varied to suit individual taste.

Gravy, without the use of flour as thickening, can be made using mushroom powder instead. Other gravy thickeners you can use are egg yolks, or canned vegetables pulverized in a blender.

Milk products are reduced in calories by exchanging whole milk at 140 calories a cup to skimmed milk at 70 calories a cup. Powdered milk also has many interesting applications.

Salads can be made more appetizing with the use of gelatin to make an aspic. There are no calories in gelatin. Salad dressings are made by the exchange of low-calorie ingredients.

For example: A boiled dressing at a value of 30 calories per tablespoon is normally made with two egg yolks, 1½ tablespoons of flour, 1½ tablespoons of sugar, 1½ tablespoons of butter, ¼ cup milk and cup of vinegar, plus seasonings. This is reduced to 9 calories per portion when the flour, sugar, butter and milk is exchanged as previously described. All dressings may be handled in this manner without sacrifice of taste. This also applies to sauces and soups.

There are those who will warn against frying and advise to limit most types of cooking to boiling and broiling when on a diet. But ours is not really a diet. We can eat fat and not get fat because we are not providing the carbohydrate hooks which the body uses to hang fat on. We understand it is actually dangerous to our health if we do not enjoy diversified foods since it will lead to compensation which, from past experience, we know will lead to overeating as well as overconsumption of sweets and starches. So we not only boil and broil but we also fry, stew, sauté, roast, steam, and pressure-cook.

Some animals at the Veno Zoo in Tokyo recently were put on diets because they had gained considerable weight. An orangutan went from 150 pounds to 242 and had to be put on one-third rations. A gorilla that puffed up to 550 pounds from 450 in one month's time was switched from sweet potatoes to milk. Signs had to be put up warning visitors not to feed the animals. They have had enough. The similarity with human weight problems is all the more apparent when you hear zoo officials explain how overweight animals tend to suffer from poor physical coordination, impaired virility, and susceptibility to disease.

Do you blame me for being thrilled when I receive success stories from my women clients? "Dear Mr. Petrie," writes one lady, "although I have not seen you for three years, I want to tell you that I am now down to 128 pounds and can still hardly believe it. I am eating well, enjoy everything, and realize now that I will never have a weight problem again."

To which we can all say "Amen."

Review of Chapter Highlights

How to change your favorite recipes, substituting for or eliminating sugar, flour, bread crumbs, and other carbohydrate ingredients. Put in their stead some of those in Appendix I that appeal to you. Use some of the health hints from abroad on page 136. How to plan some delicious low-calorie snacks for your next party.

12

How To Strengthen Your Determination
and Drive To Lose Weight

I am going to get quite personal with you in this chapter. We are going to delve beneath the surface of palates, pleasantries and pulchritude and turn the spotlight on some seldom-bared recesses of your inner thoughts.

The purpose of this venture inward is to reinforce your desire to lose weight, to make you want to be thin so earnestly that it will become the easiest thing in the world for you to accomplish.

We will be talking person to person about some serious matters as the effect of extra pounds on health and the importance of being attractive.

I will give you the secret of auto-suggestion that will make your switch to healthful eating habits practically automatic. You will reach for a cheese instead of a sweet just as if you had been doing so all your life.

Auto-suggestion is one of the most effective methods of appetite and diet control ever discovered. You will be amazed at the instant results.

A woman who had been coming to me for three weeks stepped on my office scale. "I've gained!" she cried out in surprise. "I've gained two pounds. I don't understand it. What does this mean?" "It means you have gained two pounds," I replied. What else could I say?

This woman had done well the first two weeks—losing four pounds the first week and two pounds the second. She had not lost enough to hit a valley, as is so often the case after a few weeks of successful losing. What did hit a valley was her resolve. In fact, it had just about disappeared. She needed to recharge her purpose and reset her goals. I was able to help her do this at that single session and the following week the scale proclaimed the success of our effort.

"It took a great deal of courage for me to come," confessed one food-loving woman. A four-pound gain over the Christmas holidays finally tipped the scales in my favor, she explained. Some women's resolve can be strengthened only when they court the next larger dress size. I got this particular woman to buy herself an attractive dress one size too small. It worked. In two weeks she was wearing it.

A Reminder of That Girl You Can Be

Most women are so brainwashed by their diet failures that they begin to accept themselves in their new massive, unattractive silhouette. They lose their stomach for the battle of losing weight. Resolve is nil.

"Tomorrow I am going to do something about getting back in shape." It's never *today*, when resolve is below par. One of the reasons I have captured some of my women in "before" and "after" photos is the encouragement they bring to those who feel the road ahead is too rough even to begin.

Take a look at Model B before and after. Would you have believed such a change possible, if you had been she?

What You Don't See in the Picture

What you do not see in the picture is meal after satisfying meal of such tempting dishes as coq au vin, melon prosciutto, lobster thermidor, veal fiorentina, and on and on. There is no torture on the road ahead. Tempting gourmet recipes keep Petrie "dieters" satisfied. Culinary delights keep your morale high as you whittle your weight away. Forget about the impossible diets that promised you so much and delivered so little. I want you to forget the do's and don't's that make life miserable for dieters. Instead, I want you to pamper yourself.

The road is painless and the goal is a younger, fitter, happier, prettier you. You will return to being one of those vital people who

Model B, After

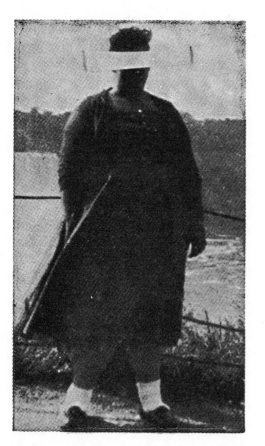

Model B, Before

keep in top physical shape. The very persons you want to notice you will react like magic to your new attractiveness. I am not quoting. Ask my thousand women clients.

The Fork in the Road

There is another road. I am going to describe it to you. But before I do I want to tell you that I have a helpful reason for doing so. You understand the "golden girl" at the end of one road open to you. Now, if you understand what is at the end of the other road open to you, I will be able to give you a simple mental exercise that will vault your resolve high above its present level and make it easier than you ever dreamed possible to carry out eating-habit changes *without painful will power*.

It may be unpleasant reading, but stay with me. It will be worth the few minutes, since it will mean you are eligible to carry out the fork-in-the-road exercise that will follow.

At the other end of the road is a corpse. She has succumbed before her years. It could have been her heart.

Heart disease is the greatest single cause of death in the United States and it plays favorites with overweight people. It also singles out those overweight people with carbohydrate-rich, sweet diets. Reporting in GP, a medical journal, Dr. Charles H. Duncan and Dr. Maurice M. Best, physicians at the University of Louisville School of Medicine, say that evidence points to blood cholesterol, a type of fat, tending to be higher in persons who receive most of their carbohydrates in the form of sugar, candy, soft drinks, pies, pastries, etc. The link between this high-serum cholesterol and premature death from coronary disease is indisputable.

It could also have been a stroke. Disease of the arteries, known as arteriosclerosis, can cause stroke as easily as coronary thrombosis. It can occur through high blood pressure, which often walks hand in hand with obesity.

It could have been her kidneys, or diabetes, arthritis or her digestive system. There is no limit to the kind of troubles obesity can bring. Chronic illness creeps up and becomes a way of life. It can start with simple overtiredness and persistent fatigue and snowball into one health crisis after another. Surgery becomes more and more necessary and less and less successful as the surgeon duels with the extra layers.

The insurance fraternity has a 50-50-50 rule of thumb. A woman of fifty who is 50 pounds overweight has a 50 percent less life expectancy. This means ten more years to go instead of 20. The quicker she takes off the weight, the fewer the years off her life. The toll is inevitable. Insurance statistics are based on that fact.

I told you it would not be a pretty story.

The Danger of Diet Pills

There is more to the tale of woe. Women who turn to diet pills are courting their own special kind of health disaster.

Recently weight-reducing pills were implicated in the deaths of six women in Oregon. The State Medical Examiner, Dr. Russell Henry, said that the women had suffered a fatal depletion of potassium in their systems as a result of taking a series of different pills. These pills contained phenobarbital, amphetamines, digitalis, thyroid vegetable laxatives and a lot of other "dynamite."

Dr. Henry's findings have led to a government investigation of diet pill companies. The American Medical Association has long decried the wholesale dispensing of diet pills by so-called obesity specialists after only superficial examination.

Digitalis is a powerful substance. So is thyroid extract. They greatly stimulate the system and step up the metabolic rate. Followed by tranquilizers and appetite depressants, they deal a double blow to the body, first whipping it to a faster pace, then slowing and dulling the processes. Repeat this daily and it is little wonder that a few weeks of such violence to the body can take its toll. The toll has been heart failure and other fatal complications.

Women have come to me in a state of physical exhaustion and bordering on mental and physical collapse as a result of a diet-pill program that has upset their glands, fractured their nerves, and dehydrated their bodies of life fluids. They are weak, short of breath, or irritable. They often perspire profusely and malodorously. They have palpitations of the heart, rash, or dizziness. Their vitality is draining away.

What a difference after a few meals such as broiled lamb chops, collard greens and salad, and a couple of high-protein, high-nutrition, low-carbohydrate, no-drug days (or daze)!

How To Harness Your Subconscious for Slimming

With the foregoing sordid details out of the way, we are now ready for that mental exercise that I promised you. It requires only a quiet room and three to five minutes of relaxed concentration. In those few minutes you will harness the vast power of your subconscious mind to propel you to slimming your figure, and "easy will do it" for you.

With one brief visual image you will neutralize much of the brainwashing to which you have been subjected by candy commercials, ice cream ads, and cake-mix billboards. You will neutralize the effect of your own emotional causes for overeating. And you will banish the discouragement of past diet failure.

Does that promise sound like a fantastic? Believe me, it is even more fantastic than you think! Much has been written about the powers of the mind but there is nothing like seeing the mind in action to appreciate the miracles that can be wrought. The women that have used auto-suggestion never stop singing its praises to me.

What Auto-Suggestion Did for a 425-Pound Woman

Mrs. S. is thirty-five years old and the wife of a department store executive. She came to me while in a state of deep depression—having put on more than 100 pounds in a period of eleven months. As a teenager she weighed between 130 and 150 pounds. After her marriage she soared to 280 pounds and progressively climbed to the 425 pounds where my chart for her began. Here is her own description of the problem and the solution.

> I was an overweight child and remained overweight into my adulthood. About ten years ago I had a nervous breakdown, started to eat even more compulsively. I have been on many diet programs, some self-imposed and some with pills, and all have failed. I never have followed through until I started auto-suggestion.
>
> How did I become aware of auto-suggestion for weight control? My dentist told me about it and I heard about you through your book on controlling weight through self-hypnotism.[1] Since I have been coming to you I have had marvelous control. I don't think about food all the time and the most important thing is that for the first time in my life I really believe that I will get down to a normal weight and stay there.

---

[1] Sidney Petrie, *How to Reduce or Control Your Weight Through Self-Hypnotism* (Englewood Cliffs, N.J.: Prentice-Hall, Inc., 1965).

She did. Inside of five months she had lost 100 pounds. The second 100 pounds took seven months. I crossed out the case at 185 pounds, with her weight still descending and Mrs. S. a happy woman.

Relaxing is nothing new, you say; you do it every night. Fine. Keep doing it. But you cannot auto-condition yourself in the sleeping state. You must seek to attain a deep state of relaxation just short of sleep.

This threshold of sleep is a fascinating state to be in. It is the threshold also to the subconscious. This is why auto-suggestion is so effective when conducted while in this state.

Early in this century the French psychologist Coué had everybody looking in the mirror and saying, "Every day in every way I am getting better and better." This might be called Western man's first attempts at self-help through auto-suggestion. The late Dr. Hornell Hart then became the father of modern auto-suggestion and gave us the term auto-conditioning to mean the improvement of our moods and attitudes through the use of auto-suggestion. He used relaxation, where Coué did not. Results were magnified manyfold.

A Visual Exercise for Effective Auto-Suggestion

Psychologists explain that the quieting of the body and the mind permits suggestions to reach deep into the subconscious without the blocking effect of an active conscious mind. When you relax physically you are better able to blank your mind. The deeper your relaxation, the better the suggestion you give yourself takes root.

A method of progressive relaxation was given to you in Chapter 8, (See pages 95 and 96). I want you to re-read one of these monologues so that you have the main steps committed to memory. When you are thoroughly relaxed, you are ready for the simple mental exercise that will strengthen your resolve to lose weight in a no-effort, operation-bootstrap way.

Here is what you do. When you are at the deepest point of your relaxation, and your mind is perfectly blank, visualize the two roads we described before. On the left is the road to obesity and ill health. On the right is the road to slenderness, personal success and good health. *You see yourself turning away from the left road and starting down the right-hand road.*

That is all there is to it. Two factors—deep relaxation and sharp visual imagery—make this exercise infallible. Practice deep relaxation. Improve your visualization. Then, when you continue to do this exercise once or twice a day for a week or so, you will have paved the way for effortless dieting, painless self-control and quick success.

Important. You cannot benefit from this simple mental exercise just by reading about it. You must put the book down and try it. Why not read the relaxation monologue again right now, then put the book down and try it.

You Can Think Yourself Thin and Attractive

There are many suggestions you can give yourself that will propel you along the road to that attractive new shape. Whatever you feel you should do, but never seemed to get the spunk or will power to carry through with, you can now do without any more holdback. Just perform the two road exercise: the left road leads to the painful existence resulting from the unwanted condition, the right road leads to the joyful existence possible through the changed conditions. You see yourself taking the right-hand road to a joyful existence.

Here are some of the changes you can bring about by performing this visual exercise in a thoroughly relaxed state:

(a) You can picture yourself overweight as you are now and on the road to getting worse, then you can picture yourself slender and on the road to getting more and more attractive. You choose the latter.

(b) You can picture yourself tired, bored, and in the doldrums; then you can picture yourself selecting the road to an energetic, vital, and dynamic life.

(c) You can see yourself wracked with fear, doubt and uncertainty; then you can picture yourself selecting the road to confidence, purpose and decision.

(d) You can see yourself a slave to bread and potatoes and headed down the road to grim obesity; and you can see yourself choose in its place the path of proteins and salads and a glorious, lithe and svelte body.

(e) You can see yourself at the crossroads of eating your gluttonous way down the road to an early grave, or eating sensible portions to lengthen your life. You choose modest dining, health and longevity.

(f) You can see yourself untidy, unkempt, and unsightly on the way to personal obscurity; and you can see yourself interested in your clothes, your coiffure and your appearance and selecting the road to friendships and popularity.

The list is endless. The power of positive thinking is not only transforming fat people into thin people, but it is transforming the "I can't" people into "I can" people, failures into successes, "milquetoasts" into leaders, and pain-wracked hypochondriacs into the effervescently healthy.

Learn to practice this visual exercise to help you acquire the motivation you need to reach your goals of beauty, health and personal happiness. A few minutes a day will increase your skill in relaxation and in visualizing and the results will begin to snowball.

How Others Can Help You

"I decided to get off ice cream and came back from shopping without that item for a change. My husband, who constantly taunts me about my weakness for it, made his usual comment about "what forty-eight delicious flavors did you buy today?" That did it. I went back out and came back with a quart of strawberry, coffee and maple walnut."

So spoke a newlywed who was fast becoming a matronly "hausfrau." Her husband's moral support was obviously less a supportive than an undermining influence.

This is so often the case in many families. The overweight person who is confronted with constant reminders such as "don't eat this" and "stop eating that" is more likely to rebel than comply.

The family may not be able to help you strengthen your drive to lose weight. Rather they can be a psychological drag on that drive. I have found that my women fare better ignoring the reactions of members of the family—spouse, children, parents, etc.—and confiding their goals instead to friends who are sympathetic because of their own similar problem.

Many women go to Take Off Pounds Sensibly (TOPS) clubs, and other weight-watching groups, and can attribute their tons of success to the strengthening of resolve that can come through "mutual assistance pacts." "Phone me next time you feel like having some candy" is strongly similar to the use of the telephone by members of Alcoholics Anonymous.

The persons most likely to help you in a reciprocal arrangement are those with which you normally have day-to-day contact—women who live nearby or who work in the same office. Share your goals, review together your progress charts, help each other with carbohydrate calorie values, exchange high-protein recipes, and discuss the art of relaxation and visual imagery to improve success for both in the practice of auto-suggestion.

If you know several women who are interested in the same goals, you can start your own club. Meet once a week to exchange ideas, compare successes, and strengthen self-confidence in ever-greater progress in the weeks ahead.

Special tip: Keep such a group confidential, especially from the negative remarks and taunts of respective families.

The Remarkable Eight-Meals-A-Day Diet

Sometimes a woman gives up because she just cannot resist snacks in between meals. I know she can *lose weight even with snacking* and so do my 1,000 other women clients. It is no reason to become discouraged about snacking. And certainly absolutely foolhardy to give it up.

I have put many women on a plan of almost constant eating to prove that they can still lose weight without giving up their frequent trips to the kitchen.

Before I reveal this remarkable program to you I want you to understand the scientific reasons why it works.

Do you know that if you were to split up a meal and eat part of it now and the rest of it a couple of hours later, that meal would be less fattening? It is absolutely true.

Experiments have shown that the tendency to gain weight is greater from the same number of calories if they are all eaten in one meal. By dividing these calories into two or more meals, the effect on increasing weight is less. Thus by taking your present three meals a day, on which you are failing to lose weight, and dividing them up into six meals or even eight meals, you are likely to see the needle on the scale begin to dip in your favor.

One pitfall, though, is the difficulty in keeping track of calories or carbohydrates where six or eight meals are involved. We tend to forget the smaller eating events. Better put a close control on this counting procedure if you embark on this eating, eating, eating program.

Every variety of animal on which it has been tried has grown more obese if forced to eat only two meals daily, even though given an ideal diet. Domestic dogs and cats are far more overweight percentage-wise than even humans in our affluent urban and suburban homes. They often grow fatter when cut down to once a day feeding. When allowed small frequent feedings of the identical food, animals, domestic or otherwise, maintain their normal weight.

Food is converted mostly into energy when frequent small meals are eaten. However, large meals can overwhelm the enzyme systems in the body. The transfer into energy is incomplete. A large portion is stored as fat.

Large meals can be disastrous to a slender figure. They can be even more disastrous when eaten in the evening, as is most often the case, when the consumption of energy begins to decline and in a few hours, during sleep, reaches its low ebb. That is when the body converts the excess to fat instead of to energy. Table 6 gives two programs for an eight-meal-a-day diet. Use the one you need now.

Eating Habit Patterns of People Who Can't Reduce

The eating habits of most people who cannot reduce follow a strikingly similar pattern. They arise in the morning with a high blood-sugar content from all of the food consumed the night before that has not been burned off, and a high resolve not to overeat. So they skip breakfast. They will even eat a very light lunch. But come dinner time, the lid is off.

It should be just the other way around. Breakfasts should be substituted—high in lasting proteins that keep you satisfied and hunger-pang free. Lunches should emphasize the proteins and nutrients—greens and other growing foods. And dinners should be much lighter than they are.

You can make the transition to this new weighted eating—heavier breakfasts and lighter dinners—by using the eight-meal-a-day routine as an interim measure. It is also an excellent way of proving to yourself that you can eat, eat, eat and still lose weight.

You need to know this. You need to be confident that there is no deprivation on the road to sustained health and maintained weight. Try it and see. You can create your own diet, using the same principle of dividing one meal into two or three or in any other manner, spreading the same calorie count over the eight meals.

You should find that the very fact you can eat this way and still lose weight is very reinforcing to your drive to reduce. In fact, admit this: It is the most reassuring moment you have ever had. What has persisted as a dream—unreachable at the end of a diet treadmill—is now closer to reality than ever before.

Eight-Meals-a-Day
Weight-Loss Diet

(A total of 1,000 calories of which 15 percent is carbohydrate)

Meal 1

½ c. strawberries
1 poached egg
coffee

Meal 2

4 oz. cr. of tomato soup
1 Ritz cracker or
1 water biscuit

Meal 3

Tuna salad made with 2 oz. of tuna
large lettuce leaf 2 sl. tomato with
lemon juice

Meal 4

Fruit Salad made with ½ orange
1 sl. water-pack pineapple
lettuce, 1 tb. Fr. dressing

Meal 5

1 sl. diet bread with 1 sl. Am.
cheese grilled with sl. of tomato

Meal 6

1 lg. tomato stuffed with 2 oz.
chopped white meat of chicken
2 chopped celery stk.
Sprinkle Parmesan cheese on
and grill

Meal 7

2 oz. cottage cheese on ½ water-
packed pear

Meal 8

D-Zerta pudding with 2
chopped walnuts and marachino
cherry

Eight-Meals-a-Day
Weight-Maintenance Diet

Meal 1

4 oz. fresh orange juice
1 fried egg
coffee

Meal 2

American cheese and one slice bacon
or 2 soybean crackers.

Meal 3

4 oz. cream of mushroom soup
1 water biscuit

Meal 4

3 oz. tuna fish salad
Tea with lemon

Meal 5

2 oz. cottage cheese or half of
pear

Meal 6

4 oz. broiled hamburger with
mushroom caps
Coffee

Meal 7

4 oz. fruit salad, lettuce, mixed
greens

Meal 8

Shrimp cocktail. Diet dessert.

Table 6

Review of Chapter Highlights

How to use the simple art of relaxation and auto-suggestions can make the switch to healthful eating habits automatic. Increase your motivation drive by reminding yourself where the ugly obesity road leads to. Choose the slenderness road in an auto-suggestion exercise. Remind yourself also of the dangers of diet pills. Choose the nutrition road to a better life. You can eat as many as eight smaller meals a day and lose weight even faster.

13

How To Make the Most of Your Best

Features

Part of the motivation of any person to want to look her best is to see tangible results for the effort. Each improvement sends the spirits soaring and sets the stage for the next improvement.

I make it a practice to compliment my clients for any modified hair style, new dress, or change in make-up that adds to their attractiveness. I am sure I am not the only one who does, and the fact that others notice too, increases their self-confidence.

Self-confidence is so important to successful slimming. It spells all the difference between losing heart or losing weight. So I would like to share with you the myriad ways in which my women have beautified themselves.

Now I am not a beautician. These tips come from those I consider the most beautiful women in the world—my slenderized clientele. They have passed their secrets on to me so that they can build up the self-confidence of those who followed them into my office.

I have compiled these beauty tips and placed them in a semblance of an orderly program in this chapter; otherwise in reading this information you might be overwhelmed and not know where to begin. I think you should begin with your best features and make yourself irresistible through them. Then bring the rest of you up a level. That is how this chapter begins.

If you were to start with your weakest links and bring them up to average, you would still be only average in attractiveness. However, by making the most of your best features you become singularly attractive.

How To Recognize Your Good Features

"Lady Republicans have big fronts and Lady Democrats have big behinds." This remark has been making the rounds, so to speak, in Washington, D.C. for so many years its origin has been lost. Do your politics show? Does your apathy show? What does show?

The full-length mirror that helped you earlier in this book can help you again, but this time you need a close friend to stand in front of it with you. If this rules out nudity, then wear leotards, or a bathing suit. But your friend is better able than you to render a critical analysis of both your good and bad features.

In lieu of a friend, I'd insist on a three-way mirror instead of the one-glass type. If you recall, the last time you stood in front of one in a dress shop, you were struck by the sight of yourself from directions usually only another person would view you. You were getting an outsider's view.

The objective view, by friend or by three-way mirror, can turn up some little known facts about yourself. You may discover that your hair is of beautiful texture and color but there is not enough of it. Were it longer, you could picture yourself doing some interesting things with it. Meanwhile, you could rely on a wig, wiglet or fall.

You may discover that although your measurements are still too large, they are in excellent proportion and that by concentrating on better posture you can overcome the lap of weight somewhat during the period you are losing pounds.

You may discover that your complexion is of that rare silk ilk that girls seek and for which they are sought after. You may discover your eyes, your legs, your bosom—through the unbiased biased mirrors or eyes of a friend.

The Many Mirrors That Reflect You

Most stage, screen and television stars were not born beautiful. They learned to create their image by building up their good points and playing down their faults. They read everything on the subject they can lay their hands on and they seek the advice of experts and specialists such as cosmeticians, hair stylists, dress designers, and dietitians.

These women become world-renowned beauties also because they use every type of mirror available to them—not just the glass kind and the eyes of friends. They use tape recorders to mirror their voice and speech. They use film takes and screen tests to depict their walk and their movements. They have learned to watch their own mannerisms as reflecting inner attitudes and emotions.

Get a tape recorder. There are good reasonably priced small ones on the market. Listen to yourself speak. Next time someone calls you on the phone, begin recording; then play it back. Your own voice can be very revealing. It may even astound you. Is it harsh, nasal, too high-pitched, too loud? Is your speech scattered with clichés or bad grammar? If so, this is a good place to begin. Some people have a good ear and by carefully listening to an admired friend with a good speaking voice, will be able to improve their own voice greatly without outside help. If further, more detailed, changes are needed, by all means consult a good speech therapist. It's worth every penny it costs and the time it takes. No new dress, slimmer figure or lovely make-up is going to impress a living soul if you don't have speech charm. Your voice may turn out to be one of your very strong features.

Mannerisms are also a dead give-away to your inner self. They can reflect inner serenity and self-assuredness or insecurity and nervousness. Most people are completely unaware of their own movements, since they are largely involuntary and also usually controlled by the subconscious. Here that trusted friend will be helpful. Urge him, or her, to be frank. Observe and make a note of unattractive mannerisms in others about you. Be increasingly aware of yourself for a few days. Are you displaying some of these mannerisms, too, such as eye-popping, mouth-stretching, tongue-biting, hand-waving, nervous fidgeting? Remember, these are not easy habits to lick. You may have been doing these things for years, very likely most of your life.

You should use the auto-conditioning mental imaging to see yourself free of unwanted mannerisms. Develop a tranquil attitude, while still retaining your natural animation. Act the model of poised self-assuredness. A good modeling course, if available, will teach you how to sit, stand, enter a room, get in and out of a car, walk, handle accessories such as gloves, handbag. The old trick of doing these things while balancing a book on your head is still as effective as it ever was. Again, an astute person can learn much by watching

TV or screen stars move and can give themselves a charm course. Grace can be acquired. It is a part of the total picture you present. Do you look ungroomed hurrying down the street or do you present a lovely coordinated image from across the room? It is an image anyone can have, if she really wants it.

How To Improve Your Image

Statesmen, politicians, and others who are interested in how they look to others employ public relations counselors to improve their image. Here again, just because the expert is not available to us does not mean we must be satisfied with what we have. We can be our own "expert."

You may be too heavy, but while you're working on weight loss stand properly, hold your head up, look people in the eye, smile frequently, look serenely interested in what's happening to your fellow man. Even if you feel down in the dumps, don't let it show. Self-control can play a large part in how you look to the rest of the world.

Read more. Improve your conversation. Develop any creative ability you may have, no matter how small. Learn to see adventure in everyday happenings. Don't let boredom, symptom of a lazy mind, overtake you. Try new creative things. How can you know you have an ability if you do not try your hand at new modes of expression?

Even your everyday tasks can be more creative. Resolve to try one new recipe a day for a week. Work on serving meals more attractively. If you hate to cook, your talent may be in gardening, interior decorating, sewing, painting, weaving, photography or some hobby. You are bound to become a more interesting person for it—not only to men, family, and friends, but to yourself, too.

Are you a loyal friend concerned with people around you? Do you believe yourself to be a silent, uninteresting person or a drag at social functions? Has it occurred to you that the whole world needs a few good listeners and that you may be one of them? I once told this to a twenty-eight-year-old lab technician who was half-way along the 80-pound road to normalcy but who was beginning to suffer from the "I'm getting too old to be married" syndrome. She listened to me, then she listened to a young doctor's problems— really listened. Three months later they were sharing those problems.

Listen the next time, instead of worrying about the impression you make. If an idea or two works its way into your mind along the way, express it briefly. But then go back to listening. No one is a bore who shows genuine interest toward others.

How about your physical profile? Do you waddle like a duck when you walk or lean forward with your neck out like an Arizona roadrunner, or maybe you slouch trying to be shorter than you are, giving your bustline a sort of concave appearance. Do you have trouble knowing what to do with your hands and do they sometimes feel like two endless swaying clock pendulums? Don't give up—this is simply where you begin to improve your image. If you can afford it and there is one available, enroll in an exercise and posture course. The beauty magazines provide a continuing source of help and advice. There are lots of people just like you, you know.

No figure looks attractive slumped on a crooked pile of vertebrae. Pose your legs properly. Learn by watching successful actresses move on stage or screen.

You may already be quite aware of what cries for improvement in yourself but have given up because the task seems insurmountable. Tackle one fault at a time. Start with one least difficult to correct. Seeing a successful result, no matter how small, will give you the encouragement you need to proceed to the next project. You may be wearing a 1950 face or a hair-do that needs updating. To my mind, correcting this can do more for a woman's level of esprit de corps than anything else.

Now as you gaze at your new reflection notice that you are already holding your head higher and are wearing a more confident and pleasant expression. But there is more work to do.

More Hints for a Skin that Glows with Health and Beauty

Aside from the more obvious physical differences between man and woman, the soft texture of the skin is one of woman's most feminine attributes. It is also one that responds to care and treatment quite readily.

Professional treatment for the skin includes such activities as skin rejuvenation, wrinkle removal, deep cleansing, cellulite treatments, electronic exercises, oxygenation, ozone activation and muscle-toning. Treatments like these are more common in Europe. But they are becoming more popular here and schools are opening to train professionals in the use of the machines and the manual techniques of facials.

Meanwhile, most women will take advantage of the countless

lotions and potions now on the market and do it themselves. From the teens on, the skin of the face and hands needs special tender care to preserve and maintain a clear complexion, firm contours and a healthy natural look. Skin care begins with cleansing. For some women this means soaps; others prefer creams. Surprisingly, the choice is not directly dependent on whether one's skin is naturally dry or naturally oily. It is a purely personal decision. A woman may want to use cleansing cream, followed by a skin freshener one day, and soap the next. She may change her cleansing methods at different times of the year, dependent on the weather. There are lotion cleansers to whisk away dirt and make-up and emulsifying creams to act as solvents on excessive skin oil. A friction effect can be had by granular cleansers which help flake off dead skin. Many of the cleansers mentioned are medicated with an anti-bacterial action that helps keep skin antiseptic. An astringent, which may prove drying for some skins, will tighten and tone the skin and close the pores. Witch hazel is the favorite of one beautiful movie actress I know. Of course, many other astringents are available.

Much of America spends its winters in overheated apartments, offices and homes. Dry heat is damaging to sensitive skins. Here are some suggestions to combat its aging effects. Open windows for part of each day. Place containers of water, and keep them refilled, on or adjacent to radiators. Keep a kettle steaming on a stove or hot plate. Acquire more house plants to help add moisture to the atmosphere.

Steaming the face is an age-old practice among women in blustery climates. Be careful not to burn yourself. Come just near enough to the jet to get the condensing vapor but not live steam.

New hair-drying equipment on the market features a face sauna which is probably a lot safer and more comfortable. If you are fortunate enough to have a steam bath or sauna in your locality, take advantage of it at least twice a month. Your skin will be cleansed and rejuvenated by these treatments.

Facial masks stimulate circulation, clear the complexion and tone the skin. In Scotland oldfashioned oatmeal is used. Mix uncooked with warm water to make a paste, and smooth it over a carefully cleaned face. Leave for ten minutes, and work off with an ice cube. Easy to use masks are available in tubes, jars and bottles that are probably more pleasant to use and just as beneficial. Eye pads dipped in witch hazel can be used while giving yourself a mask and relaxation break.

Complexion literally includes chest, shoulders, neck and even scalp, as well as the face itself. Work creams, lotions and oils in upward firm strokes from neck and throat up the face. Around the eyes, work creams in with a gentle tapping of the finger tips in toward the nose below, outward under the brows. Gently tap area along edges of the mouth and with back of fingers softly slap under chin area. Use same technique when applying a night cream. Take time to tap in and outward along upper eyelid. Use a little rotating motion and concentrate on all expression etched lines. These lines are what give a face its distinguishing character, but none of us wants to be too much of a "character."

Skin difficulties can best be cured, as your physician will advise you, by basic good health practices: proper nutrition, plenty of fresh air, rest, exercise and common-sense skin care. He may advise medicated soaps containing hexachloraphene and other healing and anti-bacterial ingredients to combat acne, too oily skin or similar problems.

For the normal skin, soaps are available which will lather and cleanse despite hardness of water (very alkaline and thus drying to the skin); cold cream or other emollient soaps with lanolin for the lady with dry skin; "soapless" cakes, differently constituted but looking like soap; deodorant soaps that combat perspiration odors, especially common among overweight people, and hypo-allergenic products for sensitive skins. French-milled soaps, fine but expensive, are firm, hard, long-lasting mild cakes, attractive in color and fragrance. Then there is the translucent variety of clear glycerine or castile soap, which is free of excessive alkali. Though expensive, it is perfect for delicate skins.

Tension can destroy beauty. It can stiffen the neck muscles and add lines to the face. Relaxing in a warm bath can be a great boon for tired, tense muscles and nerves. Allow plenty of time for this comforting ritual. A cold bath is too stimulating. A hot bath makes the pores coarse and breaks down surface blood vessels.

You may want to use a moisturizing cream in the tub after first cleansing the face. The warm, moist air will help it penetrate the face while the rest of you is being lulled and soothed in water perfumed or bubbled with foaming bath oils or any of the many other delightful adjuncts to the pleasure of the bath. Then you may want to use a body lotion from toe to throat, after a vigorous rub-down with a towel.

A final word about skin care. My women graduates know that excessive tanning ages the skin. Though most of them look and feel better with golden or bronze skins, they know when to stop and take cover. From the thirties on—face up to it—the skin just cannot take it and will need dark protective glasses, the shade from a floppy flattering beach hat or friendly umbrella, plus protective lotions or natural oils (baby oil gives no protection against the sun, contrary to popular belief). A beautiful complexion is far more "status" than an overdone tan.

A Show of Hands for Beauty

In the Orient, where there are still servants available, a woman is most often judged by her hands. The quickest relief from work-damaged hands, according to my clients, is gloves: rubber gloves for dishes and pots and gardening, night gloves over well-creamed hands for a rejuvenated, youthful hand treatment.

Creams applied externally do help. They soothe, they smooth away roughness, and they penetrate the outer layers of the skin to restore oils. In selecting hand lotions or creams, you have a personal choice. There are protective products containing silicones which shed water, soil and chemicals. There are lotions specifically for chapped, cracked skin. (These contain allantoin, collagen, pathenol and A and B complex vitamins for healing.) There are rich, creamy products for those who like massage. And there are the non-greasy liquids for quick, frequent use.

When applying hand lotion, work some in around the nails and gently push back the cuticles. In addition, pay especial care to the cuticles when preparing hands for a manicure. Don't just apply polish. Clean nails thoroughly with an oily remover and wash off. Dry and then buff the nails. Push back cuticles and apply base coat to fill in ridges for your next two or three coats. Allow ample drying time between each. Polish will adhere longer if you do. Then top with clear lacquer. Some of my clients add a clear coat nightly and say it protects nails.

How To Make Your Face Look Thinner and More Beautiful

The art of make-up was recently given the coveted recognition of a fashion award for the first time. The total look so currently in vogue now includes the face. In fashion publications, and by the few who take them literally, the face is treated as an adjunct to fashion. My women clients have gone even further. They have confided in me ways to make a round face look thinner!

You begin your face art with a foundation. Use cream or oil, if your skin tends to be dry. Cake foundation is only for oily skin. Pick a shade close to your natural skin tone. You may even find it more effective if it is a tone lighter. At night, it can be darker or dramatically lightened to suit artificial lighting and your mood. Apply with a light touch so you do not mask your natural skin tone. Correctly applied, imperfections are minimized, the complexion is enhanced and your face begins to glow with that natural look. Be sure to blend in foundation under the chin and on the neck.

How To Contour the Appearance of a Beautiful Face

There are many effects to be achieved by facial contouring. A thinner look is one. Contouring consists of shadowing and highlighting. Here are some hints for facial problem areas.

For a face too round; using a foundation about three shades darker than normal; blend shading in from ear to ear along the jaw line. Cheeks that appear too full can be lessened by shading hollow areas beneath them.

To minimize a double chin, the darker foundation is blended in from ear to ear under chin and jawline.

A too-square jaw can be softened by shading the edges of face and jaw.

A fleshy nose can be helped by using the darker foundation on both sides of the nose to give a narrower look. Under the tip of the nose and on the edge of the nostrils, it will shorten a long nose. The prominence of a high bridge is diminished by similar shading.

Highlighting with a light shade of foundation or with a special white highlighting cream can play up or correct features. This can be applied either under or over your foundation.

Highlight your chin, if receding.

Make your brows seem to arch high by highlighting just underneath. Shadows under the eyes can be obscured by using the lightener cream at the inside corner of the eye and blending outward.

To heighten cheekbones, dab highlighter from inner eye corner to middle of ear and from outer eye corner outward to upper ear tip. Fill that area in with lightener.

Hollows at temples, collar bones under lower lip, etc., can be brought forward by filling in recessed portion only.

Smile lines can be played down in similar manner.

Try one or two shadowing or highlighting techniques and live with each a day. With patience and persistence, you will soon be putting your best face forward.

Powder can freshen up foundation and impart a fragile look to the skin.

How To Make the Most of the Power of Attraction in Your Eyes

Make-up for the eyes has been in use, by men as well as the fair sex, for more than 5,000 years. Excavations of ancient cities in India, Assyria, Egypt and China inevitably uncover jars of kohl, henna and other dyes that were used. Poets through the ages have written fervently of the mystique in eyes. There is little doubt in my mind that wcmen control much of what goes on in this world through the power of their eyes. Certainly a woman in the process of slenderizing can dominate attention with her eyes and take it off other aspects of her anatomy which she does not feel are ready for that attention yet.

Your natural eyebrows are the most perfect frame for your eyes. It is simple to care for eyebrows. Merely brush them with a clean mascara brush. Instead of plucking unruly hairs, moisten them down with a dab of soap, or if you wish, trim those you consider too long. If absolutely necessary, tweeze out hairs below brow line, pulling them in the direction in which they grow.

Eyebrow make-up should be used sparingly to emphasize natural contour of the brow, and darken it if necessary. You may use an automatic or wooden pencil, cake brush-on, cream brush-on or liquid, using the same shade as hair, or one shade darker. To de-emphasize brows, use one shade lighter. Apply in short, wispy strokes. Keep the natural look intact.

Accessories to the eyes include shadow in enchanting arrays of shades and iridescent colors as well as golds and silvers, eyelashes "au naturelle" or frankly false eyeliners that dramatize "the windows of the soul," and mascara.

Shadow can be worn day and night to enhance the color, shape and mystery of the eyes. It comes in stick, powder, cream and cake form. Of the many shades available, choose one lighter than the eyes to intensify their color.

Apply your shadow up and outward on an angle, with most of it concentrated on the lid, if your eyes are heavy-lidded. The eye, with less recessed area when open, looks its best when shadow is applied outward and down over the lid with maximum concentration above, not on, the eyelid itself.

If your eyelids are darkly pigmented or, if they are pink-toned, first cover with foundation before you apply shadow. To define the crease in the eyelid use taupe, brown or purple blue to emphasize the area, winging out as you go. Highlighting can be done to bring out the brow bone, to accent the eyelid and enlarge the eye. Blend the whitener over the whole eyelid.

To elongate the eye, dab some white on the outside corner, or apply a touch along the bottom lid to make the eyes appear larger.

Eyeliner defines, reshapes and enlarges the eyes, as well as makes them more expressive. These come in liquid, cake and pencil. Colors are on the market, as well as the usual black, brown and blue. Experiment on what flatters you most for day or evening wear.

Apply eyeliner with a narrow line at inner corner of the upper lid and paint close to lashes, since this adds to their apparent length. Widen the line as you move out toward the edge of the lashes—or beyond to widen the eye. Get varied and exotic effects with the thickness and tilt of the line. Keep it simple for day wear. Evenings, go dramatic.

The lashes can be artfully darkened and thickened with mascara or by the use of false eyelashes. Both take time and art to apply, but do much to beautify the eyes. There are cake, cream, brush-on and roll-on mascaras, as well as lash-lengtheners, a creamy mascara with fibers blended in.

Black and brown are most effective for daytime, and colors more attractive for after five. On special occasions, tip with gold and silver for additional eye allure.

Remove mascara with special pads that are kind to your skin. Recommended too, is a magnifying mirror for all application of make-up, to assure a smooth, finished look.

The most popular artificial lashes are full length, of a single thickness, and follow the natural contours of the eye. As many as three sets on the top lid and one on the bottom are in vogue for the striking few. There are double lashes available for evening wear and corner lashes for achieving special eye illusions.

Lashes should be feathered and sized to fit your eyes. Surgical glue does a good holding job, but use very little and press gently into place with a tweezer or with a tissue or cotton-covered pick.

Remove excess glue before putting them away. Apply these lashes after eye make-up is on and when lids are dry.

Rouge adds the blush of youth to complexions, dramatizes the eyes and is a helpful camouflage when applied artfully. Its color should harmonize with other make-up. You may choose cream, dry or liquid rouge. If your face is too narrow, carry your rouge straight back from mid-cheek to the line of your hair. If too wide, place rouge at an upswept angle, from mid-cheek to outer eye. Blend rouge carefully into foundation. Do not place below cheekbones or closer to nose than mid-cheek.

You are now ready to turn your eyes on the world—the eyes of an alluring, youthful woman.

Lips That Tell a Story of Beauty

As expressive perhaps as the eyes are the lips. Lipstick is used by 98 percent of American women, not only for its obvious beautifying of the lips, but to protect and soothe.

Good lipstick is made of mineral and vegetable oils and waxes, and is never greasy or tacky. The light shades now in style are flattering to most women. Colors should blend with your natural skin tones, with rouge, nails, or with the colors you wear. Dramatic contrasts are fine for special effects, but generally today women do not care to have their lips "cry with color." Try blending two shades for a natural look.

Experiment with glosses either under or over your lip coloring. Use a lipstick brush for an even line, though you may attain a more natural effect without it. It is best not to alter your natural lip line unless there are irregularities.

Lipstick can be used to emphasize good features and play down imperfections. For example: Use a darker shade on top, if the bottom lip is heavy. Use a straighter line on the lower lip to avoid an unhappy expression. You might try an upsweep at the corners for a Mona Lisa look.

Your Coiffure Allure

There's nothing lovelier than unbound hair shining in the sun, streaming in the wind. One has to decide whether the current look flatters one or whether to buck the tide.

The kindest care you can give your hair, unless it is oily, is to brush it daily from scalp to end of hair length. Go against the direction of hair growth; that is, from back to front. Brushing promotes health for the scalp as well as for the hair Use a natural bristle brush for best results.

Although brushing helps keep hair and scalp clean, regular shampoos are a "must." Dry hair, of course, should not be washed so frequently. If your hair is excessively dry, massage warm oil, such as castor, into the scalp. Preferably do it the night before and cover while sleeping. Even those with oily scalp conditions might care to do this two or three times a year for a lustrous sheen.

When washing (and try to avoid shampoos made with detergents) suds at least twice and rinse thoroughly. A famed European salon washes its customers' hair with a few drops of shampoo mixed with the white of an egg. You know me—I plug proteins inside and out. In previous chapters I have listed a few more high-protein foods for the hair.

Wet or damp hair, of course, can be set and retain its shape better than dry hair. Setting lotions add body to the hair and protect coiffures against moisture in the air. Hair sprays keep hair well groomed. However, overspraying can make one's hair look wiglike.

Whether you end up with curls or swirls or a sleek, smooth style, permanents give body to fine hair. Home permanents are quite effective, but some women will trust only their hairdresser. It is an exacting technique. Types of permanents include pincurl for casual styling; rod permanents for longer hair, longer-lasting waves; end curl for bangs, touch-ups; roller permanents to give body for smooth styling.

One in every three women colors her hair. Today hair coloring can be so natural looking that it is inexcusable to have harsh or obviously colored-looking hair. Permanent hair coloring penetrates the hair shaft to lighten or to darken it.

Skillful amateurs can do it themselves with hair color baths and color penetrating shampoos in one step. Touch-ups are necessary every few weeks. Semi-permanent hair colorings last through four or more shampoos.

Finishing Fashion Touches

Fashion has been, for the last decade, on the side of those with something to hide, and it may continue so for a while longer. Belts and sashes at the natural waist will make you glad you live in a shrinking world. There are time-honored hints for the heavy, while you are getting back into shape. For the tall and heavy, wear V-necks, one-piece shifts, narrow belts, long gloves, tailored suits, nonbulky fabrics and soft, solid colors. Flattering are vertical stripes, simple jewelry, large handbags, shoes without fussy details.

Shorter women look their best in simple styles, matching separates, long sleeves, self-belts, slightly flared skirts, hats with tall crowns.

If nature has been generous to you above the waist, don't wear tight sweaters, or ruffles or bright colors; but wear sleeveless blouses that are dark, man-tailored and of smooth material. V-necklines, again, are just right for you. If you're too small on top, just reverse this.

Other problem areas such as heavy hips can be camouflaged by flared skirts, overblouses, A-lines, flat, wide pleats, and by leaving pants to the men. Minimize a large waist by avoiding belts or using self-belts, covering up with Chanel-type jackets and gathered skirts. Too narrow shoulders can be slightly padded. Horizontal stripes, wide collars and puffed sleeves will also add to shoulder width. Shoulders too broad need the opposite.

Heavy legs should be sheathed in subdued, seamed stockings and narrow, heeled pumps. Wear flared skirts of a discreet length.

Overweight may lead to an over-corseted body, but as you slim, the popular power-net underpinnings will help you present a trimmer appearance. You may get to the point of discarding girdles, but make sure your tummy muscles are firm enough first and you've formed the habit of using them and buttock muscles to form a natural girdle. If you never achieve this, do wear a comfortable but slimming foundation or your clothes, no matter how carefully chosen, will never look right.

Have enough beauty tips to keep you busy? Fine, now let's get back to food.

Review of Chapter Highlights

How to have your friends help your mirror to analyze the good points of your appearance. How to use beauty aids to emphasize them. Include your voice and mannerisms in the self-analysis, so you can improve your whole image. How to apply facial masks, skin lotions and creams to work their natural magic. Using make-up constructively and effectively for a new, natural and more attractive you. How eyes, lips, face, chin, hair get the treatment they require for a more beautiful **you**. The right fashions for you make your transformation to more graceful beauty complete.

14

How To Stay Slim Eating and Drinking at Restaurants, Parties and Barbecues

The low-carbohydrate, high-protein way of life permits you to enjoy the pleasures of eating at their best while you remain delightfully slender.

"How do you do it" says a matron to a model in a diet product commercial on TV. The answer, says the young pretty, is diet bread. Well, the answer for my 1,000 slender women clients is duck a l'orange, veal cutlet Holstein, broiled swordfish steak, and roast prime sirloin of beef.

How do they do it? By eliminating, or sharply limiting the bread—diet or otherwise—and the potatoes and the sweets. In short, by counting their carbohydrate calories, they can count on enjoying the good life.

Don't misunderstand me. You cannot lose weight living it up on gourmet dinners and party drinking. But you can maintain your weight doing it, and this chapter tells you how.

Two, Three and Four Drinks before Dinner?

Shall I mix us martinis before we begin? You can enjoy two, or three, or more if you like. Nobody is counting. The reason: there is hardly a trace of carbohydrate in gin or vodka.

That is the secret to remaining youthfully slender as you drink. No carbohydrates. What, then, is allowable, and what is off limits?

We mentioned martinis. You use a small amount of vermouth

with the gin or vodka. Usually it is dry vermouth. There is only one
carbohydrate calorie in one ounce of dry vermouth. But were you to
use sweet or Italian Vermouth, it jumps to 14 carbohydrate calories
per ounce. This can add up in the normal hour of cocktailing. And
the few carbohydrate excesses can add up during the day. Then
they can multiply when protein and fat combine with these carbohydrate hooks to hang fat on you.

The permissive moral: Drink carbohydrate-less liquor, if you
drink. And the choice is immense. About the only beverages that are
taboo are beer (except perhaps the new low-carbohydrate brands)
sweet wines, sweet cordials, and the mixed drinks or cocktails that
include sugar, sugared mixes or other off-limit carbohydrate ingredients.

This means a green light for scotch, rye, rum, gin, cognac, vodka,
bourbon, dry wine, and brandy as far as affecting unwanted pounds
is concerned.

You can have any of the afore-mentioned straight, mixed with
water on the rocks, or mixed with club soda.

Let us take it from A to Z. Applejack is fine, as are most brandies,
even apricot. Chablis is a dry wine. French champagne is dryer
than most domestic dry varieties. Stay away from the Creme de
Cocoa, Creme de Menthes and similar sweetish cordials. Hard cider
is a little too hard on the carbohydrate count (seven carbohydrate
culprits to a six-ounce glass).

A gin rickey is on the border line. That means a one-drink limit.
When others order manhattans, make yours scotch manhattans or
dry manhattans. Rob Roys are fine. Rum is yes, Jamaica or bacardi.
Dry wines include chianti, claret, burgundy, and some of the other
red wines. Also chablis, Moselle, Rhine and some of the white wines.
I said A to Z. Stay away from zombies; their 100-carbohydrate
calories will make you look like a fat one in time.

How To Enjoy Eating Out Without Conscience Pangs

Eating out is one of America's favorite pastimes. In a large me-
tropolis, a list of restaurants sounds like rollcall at the United Nations. Overweight or underweight, we are an adventuresome people
at the dinner table.

You can continue to be adventuresome and still remain lithesome.
Fortunately the world's most enjoyable foods are high in protein
and low in carbohydrates. With few exceptions, as in the Italian

pastas and Chinese noodle dishes, eating out can be a permissive adventure.

I would like to take the typical dinner menu from a good restaurant (Table 7) and suggest how to order. We will order from the tempting array of foods that will benefit your slimming figure.

Appetizers

Pâté Maison is chopped liver. It gets my vote for being highest in valuable nutrients, lowest in carbohydrate calories. Commendable choices, too, are the clams, shrimp, escargots (snails) and sturgeon; these seafood items are all rich in minerals and have barely a trace of carbohydrates. Clams Casino are whole clams topped with bacon; fine. Not so fine are the minced clams, which are mixed with bread crumbs (but do not happen to be on this menu). While your conventional diet friends order the grapefruit, tomato juice, supreme of fruit, or melon, about the only appetizer you might avoid as a fat builder is the eggplant provençale.

Soups

Say yes to the onion soup and put all the grated cheese you want in it, but dip the spoon in past that piece of toast floating in it. Consommé is fine, but vichyssoise is potato soup. The day I ate at this restaurant the potage du jour happened to be Manhattan clam chowder. I ordered it, but ate my way around the potatoes.

Entrees

Sole, scallops, lobsterettes, and scampi are great seafood dishes, almost totally without carbohydrate calories. Watch out for the frogs' legs sauté Meunière; depending on the chef, they can be thickly coated in a batter. Crêpes of seafood cardinal are not for us; crêpes are pancakes. Stuffed shrimp and crabmeat Maryland are borderline. Shrimp and crabmeat are tops, but that Maryland may ring in a bread or potato stuffing, depending on the chef.

Order the duckling, broiled spring chicken, coq au vin, or capon. But avoid the stuffed breast of chicken Cordon Bleu or the Cornish hen stuffed with wild rice. In each case, the word stuffing is the tip-off—bread or rice, it spells stuffing for you as much as the bird. Breaded veal cutlet has the bread on the outside, which is almost as bad. Order instead the scalopini of veal with mushrooms. Of course, it is green light on the filet mignon (if it is sliced, you'll eat less), lamb chops, and sirloin steak. This restaurant, like most others,

A TYPICAL RESTAURANT DINNER MENU

Appetizers

Pâté Maison	Supreme of Fruit	Sturgeon à la
Marinated Herring	Egg à la Russe	Suisse
Shrimp Cocktail	Escargots Bourguignonne	Tomato Juice
Cherrystone Clams	Shrimp	Eggplant pro-
Melon in Season	Baked Clams Casino	vençale
		½ Grapefruit

Soups

French Onion Soup   Potage du Jour   Consommé   Vichyssoise

Entrees

Filet of Sole, Lemon Butter
Frogs' Legs Sauté Meunière
Long Island Bay Scallops en Brochette or Sauté
Broiled Imported Lobsterettes, Drawn Butter
Baked Clams Casino
Broiled Scampi Rendezvous
Crêpes of Seafood Cardinal
Stuffed Shrimp au Crabmeat Maryland
Roast L. I. Duckling Bigarade
Whole L. I. Duckling Flambé for Two
Broiled Spring Chicken American
Breaded Veal Cutlet Parmagiana or Holstein
Stuffed Breast of Chicken Cordon Bleu
Coq au Vin Berichone
Sliced Breast of Capon en Broccoli, au Gratin
Roast Boneless Cornish Hen Stuffed w. Wild Rice
Scalopinii of Veal, Maderia Sauce w. Mushrooms
Sliced Filet Mignon, Bordelaise
Broiled Lamb Chops Vert Pre
Broiled Prime Sirloin Minute Steak
Broiled Prime Sirloin Maitre d'Hotel
Broiled Prime Filet Mignon

Desserts

Peach Melba	Coupe aux Marrons	French Ice Creams
Bisquit Tortoni	Home Made Pies	Parfait Maison
Cherries Jubilee	Baked Alaska	Crepe Suzette (for two)

Coffee   Tea   Milk   Coffee Espresso

Table 7

serves salad with a choice of dressings, baked potato, and a vegetable. Ignore the potato as if it were not there. Taste the vegetable if it looks starch just to satisfy your taste-bud curiosity, and of course enjoy the salad with any dressing.

Desserts

Here is where the boom is lowered with a crash. There is not a single dessert listed that should interest you. But all is not lost. The waiter will be glad to bring you an order of cheese, or jello, or one of the fruit appetizers that appear on the menu: grapefruit, melon or fruit cocktail.

You have enjoyed a gourmet dinner in the finest tradition with no setback to your slender silhouette and certainly no deprivation of nourishment whatever. You will be able to do likewise at most good restaurants. Even at Italian restaurants there are a number of non-pasta appetizers, like melon prosciutto; there is onion soup instead of minestrone, and entrees like scampi, veal scalopini, chicken cacciatore—all high in protein and free of the dough that characterizes much Italian food, but you still have an excellent choice.

Eating out, guided along the same low-carbohydrate, high-protein lines as eating in, can perpetuate your youthful figure as you enjoy one of life's exciting adventures.

Some Interesting Attitudes of My Clients

Here is how one of my women clients reacted to it all:

> This has been one of the pleasantest, most gratifying experiences of my life. Previously, the many times I dieted, I became irritable, suffered headaches as the day went on, and was extremely difficult to live with.
>
> Now my disposition seems to be permanently improved, my attitude positive, despite the fact that I am eating far less than ever. All this has taken place during a period when I attended more parties than usual and ate at many fine restaurants.

At the time she wrote this, this fifty-year-old businesswoman had come to me a couple of months before, weighing 190 pounds. She lost weight at a regular rate of two pounds a week. The last time I saw her she was at 146 and still enjoying herself as she continued to lose.

A thirty-seven-year-old bookkeeper who used to gain weight on a hunger diet of melba toast and carrot sticks said, "I never realized that a diet could include clams casino, hollandaise sauce, and whipped cream and be so successful."

A twenty-seven-year old secretary who had lost 67 pounds and was on a maintenance diet told me, "I am eating more now and am more satisfied with food than I can ever remember." Her weight held fast at 130.

This from a school teacher who reduced from 188 to 140 and after leaving me continued to lose: "I never realized that food can be so tasty and succulent. I used to eat all the glop in the world."

Party Snacks and Canapés That Are Fat-Less Fun

I enjoy parties and eating at parties is an important part of the fun. I maintain my own weight at a proper level or I certainly would not be in any shape to counsel others. When I give a party, I enjoy preparing high-protein, low-carbohydrate party snacks and canapés. Let me share a few of my favorites with you.

Some folk like to put cheese on small crackers, or ham. I take cubes of cheese and cubes of ham and pin them together with a toothpick. No crackers. They are always a hit.

Popular among the party set are triangles of bread toasted on one side with American cheese and bits of sliced bacon. I put the cheese and bacon on pieces of celery stalks. No bread.

Or I broil the bacon, then roll it with an American cheese slice in a cabbage or lettuce leaf and serve it.

I make any number of dips and instead of dipping with crackers, my guests use green pepper or tomato wedges or raw cauliflower or cabbage leaves. Try my chicken liver pâté this way (I mix the cooked chicken livers with hard-boiled eggs and fried onions).

Eggs are their own canapés. When they are hard-boiled, cut in half, take out the yolks, mash them, mix them with your favorite foods and put them back in the white halves. I make deviled eggs with bacon, with cheese and with many types of shellfish. Remember to moisten with mayonnaise or catsup.

Cocktail frankfurters and little meatballs can always be found on my party tables, kept hot in casseroles and surrounded by plenty of colorful toothpicks that add nary a carbohydrate calorie. And you can say the same for their skewered morsels.

I sometimes serve mushroom caps that you can pop into your mouth sans cracker or toothpick. I cut off the stems and chop them with celery and onion, season them with salt and pepper and stuff back into the caps. A touch of grated cheese and butter goes on top and then I broil them. Always a conversation piece. You can do a number of inventive things with mushroom caps and hardly ever miss. Even served broiled au naturelle, the platter is usually one of the first to be emptied. Incidental intelligence: mushrooms are low in total calories, devoid of carbohydrate calories, and quite nutritious.

The fun list is endless. Lobster chunks, salami cubes, sardines, chicken squares, steak chunks, shrimp, herring, salmon—they all deserve an invitation to your non-fattening cocktail parties.

Do not invite bread or crackers. Use anything else you can think of. If it is not portable by toothpick, use lettuce leaves, cabbage leaves, celery stalks, green peppers, cucumbers, tomato slices or egg-white halves.

Since we have a somewhat permissive attitude toward permanent eating regimens, so that they remain permanent, I would like to give you one cracker that you might use occasionally when your favorite spread just demands a cracker. Soybean crackers are quite tasty and contain far less carbohydrates than other crackers.

You have heard me mention soybeans before in this book. There are soybean flours, milk substitutes and other soybean products. The protein in soybean is of a good nutritional quality. It contains all of the essential amino acids and contributes beneficial amounts of vitamins and minerals to the diet.

I thought I better remind you especially of the soybean cracker. If I left you with the feeling that something like crackers were totally forbidden I would be setting the stage for your breaking the ban some day. That would be falling into the diet trap all over again.

Nothing is banned, only limited. Even those fattening carbohydrates ar not banned. They, too, are only limited, with 15 percent as the best figure for your best figure.

Salads for Festive Occasions

Every party buffet can be proud of its salads and salad molds. They decorate the table and at the same time provide tasty, healthful and refreshing eating. Start with the basic green salad, using a mixture of iceberg, romaine and endive lettuce. A few raw spinach leaves, a bunch of watercress, or some onion grass from outside your

porch door is always a zest-adder. You might give your guests a
choice of dressings.

Then on to the mixed family-type salads, with tomato wedges
added and sliced peppers and radishes. Bring in the sliced cucumbers, chopped onions, and celery chunks if your pleasure so
dictates, and the garlic, too.

The famous Caesar salad may have to take a back seat to some of
the other favorites, unless you are willing to add the cheese but
forgo the bread squares.

You are better off with the cole slaws and cucumber salads; the
grapefruit, peas, peach and other types of fruit salad; and the cottage cheese and yogurt salads.

The tangy highlight of many a luncheon party is the aspic. This is
made by dissolving gelatin in water, or using consommé stock. Flavorings include lemon juice, chili sauce, and salt; let cool and
thicken. It can carry the tomato flavor or the tang of lime, apple,
orange, etc.

It can be placed in any shape mold and used to encircle shrimp,
lobster, crabmeat, tuna, salmon or other seafood. It can embrace
chicken, ham, tongue or turkey salad. Or be the crowning glory of
any original creation. Low calories, low carbohydrates, high nutrition, and great fun.

How To Enjoy Barbecues and Weddings Without Adding Even Ounces of Unwanted Weight

Like eating out, eating outdoors has become one of America's
favorite pastimes. Steak, broiling in the late afternoon, is a charac-
teristic aroma of suburbia. Even apartment dwellers place miniature
barbecues on balconies to glean the tang of outdoor cooking. Now
the barbecue is being used increasingly for other meals, with Dad
rising early to prepare wake-up breakfasts of tantalizing tidbits.

Every meat that even hit the charcoal heat is slenderizing. The
sizzling steak, grilled chops, broiled burgers are all on your list of
eat-all-you-want foods. So are the rotisserie roasts, fried chicken,
and savory ribs.

Instead of wrapping potatoes in foil, though, why not grill some
tomato wedges. Sprinkle some cheese on them for that extra touch.
Or broil some mushrooms. I don't say that you should encroach on
Dad's domain but if you prepare them, I am sure he will be willing
to make room on the grill and you will have a chance to praise him
for how well they turned out.

Just don't let me catch you wrapping that white doughy stuff around the hot dogs or hamburgers. The price you pay for holding them more easily can be years off your life. A paper plate and a plastic fork that you can toss in the garbage are far preferable to a carbohydrate roll that you may carry around with you the rest of your life.

What about parties and weddings, where the choice of menu is out of your control—do you starve? Of course not. No one is insulted if you do not serve yourself to a particular item like potatoes or bread. You can eat a little of this or a lot of that.

One young lady that I knew to be a prolific partygoer, held back somewhat on her social rounds during her period of weight loss. I was curious how she made out in holding herself at the 135 pounds she was when she left me. Then I received a letter from her saying: "Dear Mr. Petrie: Although I haven't seen you for three years I want to tell you that I am now down to 128 pounds and can still hardly believe it. I am eating well and enjoy everything and realize now that I will never have a weight problem again."

What happens at a wedding when the cake is served. Do you pass it up? Well, I have a surprise for you. I say eat it. Weddings are few and far between for the average person and participating in the beautiful tradition is far more important than other considerations. I don't say you will like the cake. It may taste insipid and sickly sweet to you. You may leave most of it on your plate. But, remember, there are no iron-clad rules. This is not a diet. It is instead a way of life. So are weddings and wedding cakes. And after all, you did not eat the rice; you threw it.

To the Beauteous Reader of This Book Whom I Wish I Knew

I have been talking to you all of these pages as if you were one of my 1,000 women clients. I have given you all of the information that I have given them and some that they have given me. I have seen them all grow slimmer, and younger, and certainly more beautiful. It is frustrating to me not to be able to see your waistline diminish and the light of youth grow brighter in your eyes.

Still it is rewarding to know that there are now additional thousands who have stepped off the dreaded diet treadmill and are losing weight the permanent low-carbohydrate high-protein way that is a pleasure.

It is gratifying, too, to know that thousands of women may have given up dangerous diet pills that can reduce their purse, and their health, as rapidly as their weight and which at this moment are under Congressional investigation.

It is gratifying that many will write me, as do my clients. I can then pass on your experiences so that they may benefit others. Speaking of letters, this one came in today. "Since I have been following your way of eating everything wonderful has happened to me. I am able to wear a size 10 dress. My skin has cleared up and I have never felt as vital and alive as I do now."

Before we part, how about a cup of coffee together? I enjoy a good cup of coffee, don't you? The water's up. I always make sure the container is absolutely clean and the water cold and fresh. The water should contact the coffee only once to taste its best, so I use the drip method. It extracts the heart of the flavor from the coffee bean and carries it pure and uncontaminated to your cup. Also the coffee should never be boiled once it is brewed. Now it's ready. Isn't that good? I call it a wonderful, steaming, aromatic beverage with heart and soul and body. A danish, or doughnut with it, would be out of place. Right? (You now know it is.)

Review of Chapter Highlights

How to enjoy drinking without weight penalty at parties by sticking to low-carbohydrate cocktails and liquor. How to select the right canapes and snacks. Enjoy eating at the finest restaurants without conscience pangs by learning to select high-protein and nutritious appetizers, soups, entrees, salads and desserts. A slice of wedding cake doesn't necessarily cause you concern for added weight.

Appendix I

Selected Recipes for Weight Control
(Entrees, Vegetables, Salads, and Desserts)

The following recipes have been selected for their high-enjoy-ment value, and low-carbohydrate value. Each recipe lists its carbo-hydrate calorie count (the fattening factor), and also the total calorie count for your general guidance in controlling your calorie intake for a day.

ENTREES

TOTAL CALORIES PER PORTION: 375
CARB. CALORIES PER PORTION: 28

Spicy Steak Strips

1 tsp. ginger	2 tsp. beef stock
2 lbs. sirloin or round steak, ½ inch thick	2 c. hot water
	1 tbs. red wine vinegar
2 tbs. butter	1 tbs. arrowroot
2 tsp. worcestershire sauce	1 tbs. cold water
1 tsp. chili powder	2 tbs. red wine
¼ tsp. garlic powder	3 tbs. instant minced onions
3 tbs. water	

Cut steak into two-inch strips. Brown lightly in heavy frying pan in butter. Add chili powder, ginger, and garlic powder. Stir rehydrated onions into browned meat. Dissolve beef paste in hot water and pour over meat. Add vinegar. Cover and simmer until meat is tender, about 40 min. Mix arrowroot with cold water and stir into steak. When sauce is thickened, add wine. Garnish with parsley. Makes 6 servings.

TOTAL CALORIES PER PORTION: 427
CARBOHYDRATE CALORIES PER PORTION: 16

London Broil

1½ lb. flank steak	1 tsp. salt
1 tbs. tomato paste	⅛ tsp. pepper
1 c. hot water	2 tsp. chopped parsley
1½ tsp. garlic salt	2 tbs. salad oil
¼ c. wine vinegar	

Score flank steak well. Combine tomato paste with hot water; add garlic salt and stir. Add vinegar, pepper and salad oil, stirring well. Pour over steak and let marinate several hours at room temperature, turning steak several times. Drain steak. Broil, about 5 to 7 minutes each side, basting with marinade. Heat remaining marinade and pour over steak. Makes 4 servings.

TOTAL CALORIES PER PORTION: 470
CARBOHYDRATE CALORIES PER PORTION: 10

Steak au Poivre

1½ lb. sirloin steak	salt
1 tbs. whole black peppercorns	¼ c. brandy
1 tbs. olive oil	

Let meat stand at room temperature about 1 hr. Crush peppercorns with rolling pin. Press pepper firmly into both sides of steak. Heat olive oil. Pan-broil steak 8 to 10 minutes on each side for medium rare. Season with salt and place on warm platter. Pour brandy into pan. When sauce bubbles pour over steak. Makes 4 servings.

TOTAL CALORIES PER PORTION: 635
CARB. CALORIES PER PORTION: 14

Chicken Livers Stroganoff

1 lb. chicken livers	1 tsp. chicken stock base
¼ c. butter	½ c. hot water
2 tbs. instant minced onions	1 c. sour cream
2 tbs. water	⅛ tsp. thyme
1 tsp. arrowroot	1 tbs. sherry
1 tbs. powdered mushrooms	1 tsp. parsley

Wash livers, cut in two and brown in butter for about 5 min., turning frequently. Meanwhile, rehydrate the onions in water. Remove livers from pan; add onions and cook for 3 or 4 minutes, but do not brown. Stir in arrowroot. Combine mushrooms, chicken stock, and hot water. Add to onions. Stir in sour cream, herbs. Add chicken livers and sherry. Heat thoroughly but do not boil. Makes 4 servings.

TOTAL CALORIES PER PORTION: 343
CARB. CALORIES PER PORTION: 20

Calves Liver Supreme

1 ¼ lb. calves liver, thinly sliced   ⅛ tsp. oregano
5 tbs. butter   ⅛ tsp. parsley
6 tbs. garlic wine vinegar

Cut liver into serving-size pieces. In heavy frying pan melt 1 tbs. butter.
Saute liver quickly to retain juices, turning to brown both sides. Add
spices, remaining butter and vinegar to drippings in pan. Heat to boiling,
stirring well. Pour over liver. Makes 4 servings.

TOTAL CALORIES PER PORTION: 675
CARB. CALORIES PER PORTION: 10

Gourmet Guinea Hen

4 1-lb. guinea hens   ½ tsp. pepper
4 cloves garlic, split   ¼ c. butter
4 tsp. thyme leaves   ½ c. lemon juice
1 tsp. seasoned salt   ¼ tsp. paprika
1 tsp. salt

Preheat oven to 450°. In each hen, place 1 clove garlic, ½ tsp. thyme,
¼ tsp. seasoned salt, ¼ tsp. salt, ⅛ tsp. pepper. Make sauce: Combine ½ c.
butter with the lemon juice, paprika, remaining thyme, stir well. Heat
some of remaining butter in medium skillet, brown hens on all sides,
adding more butter if needed. Arrange hens in roasting pan, brush with
basting sauce. Roast about 40 minutes or until browned. Makes 4 servings.

TOTAL CALORIES PER PORTION: 780
CARB. CALORIES PER PORTION: 60

Duckling à L'orange

4 to 5 lb. duckling   3 whole peppercorns
2 unpeeled oranges, quartered   ½ c. butter
1 clove garlic, chopped   ¼ c. burgundy
1 tsp. salt   ½ c. orange marmalade

Preheat oven to 425°. Stuff duckling cavity with orange quarters, garlic
salt and peppers. Place duckling breast side up in shallow roasting pan.
Brush top with butter. Pour burgundy over duckling; roast uncovered
30 minutes. Reduce oven temp. to 375°; roast 40 min. basting twice with
drippings. Turn over on breast; roast 20 min. Turn back again; roast 30
min., basting with drippings. Spread duckling with orange marmalade;
roast 10 min. longer. Makes 6 servings.

TOTAL CALORIES PER PORTION: 415
CARB. CALORIES PER PORTION: 10

Chicken Chasseur

2 lb. broiler cut up	½ c. dry white wine
2 tbs. butter	½ c. tomato sauce
¼ tsp. pepper	½ c. sliced mushrooms
¼ tsp. onion powder	2 tsp. chervil
2 tsp. chicken stock base	

Brown chicken in butter; season with pepper. Combine onion powder, chicken stock base, wine, tomato sauce, mushrooms, and 1 tsp. chervil. Pour over chicken. Cover and bake for about 30 min. in a 350° oven. Uncover and bake for 10 min. more to brown well. Sprinkle with remaining chervil. Makes 4 servings.

TOTAL CALORIES PER PORTION: 825
CARB. CALORIES PER PORTION: 10

Chicken Oregano

3–4 lb. broiler, quartered	2 tsp. oregano
½ c. lemon juice	½ c. olive oil
2 tbs. chopped parsley	½ tsp. salt
1 clove garlic, chopped	Dash pepper

In small bowl, combine lemon juice with remaining ingredients. Brush chicken on both sides with lemon juice mixture. Place on broiler pan skin side down. Broil 6 inches from heat, 15 min.; brush now and then with lemon juice. Turn; broil 15 to 20 minutes longer continuing to brush with lemon juice mixture until crisp. Makes 4 servings.

TOTAL CALORIES PER PORTION: 540
CARB. CALORIES PER PORTION: 15

Geschnetzeltes (Veal Dish from Switzerland)

2 medium onions chopped	½ tsp. salt
½ stick butter	½ tsp. pepper
2 sm. c. sl. mushrooms	Dash all-purpose seasoning
2 lb. veal for scallopini	½ c. white wine
	¼ pt. sour cream

Melt butter in skillet until lightly browned. Add onions and cook until golden. Toss in drained mushrooms and seasonings. Cook until golden. Add the veal to the skillet and cook gently until tender. This takes about 10 to 15 minutes. Add the white wine and let simmer. Remove from heat and stir in sour cream. Serves six.

TOTAL CALORIES PER PORTION: 240
CARB. CALORIES PER PORTION: 10

Savory Cheese Custard

4 eggs	2 slices boiled ham
4 tbs. milk	2 tbs. finely sliced leeks (whites
½ tsp. salt	only)
1 c. Jarlsberg Norwegian cheese, grated	1 to 2 tbs. butter

Mix eggs lightly together with milk and salt. Heat butter in a skillet, pour in egg mixture, sprinkle cheese over this and decorate with chopped ham and leeks. Cover the skillet and cook over medium heat for 5 to 6 minutes, until top is firmly set and risen and bottom is golden brown. Serves 4 to 5.

TOTAL CALORIES PER PORTION: 425
CARB. CALORIES PER PORTION: 8

Poulet Grillé au Naturel

One 2½ lb. broiling chicken	2 tbs. minced shallots or scal-
2 tbs. butter	lions
1 tbs. cooking oil	½ c. beef or chicken bouillon
Salt	

Preheat broiler. Dry chicken. Melt butter with cooking oil and brush chicken all over. Arrange skin side down in shallow broiling pan. Brush with butter and oil every 5 minutes; at the end of 15 minutes, baste, sprinkle with salt and turn chicken skin side up. Continue broiling, basting every 5 minutes for another 15 minutes or until drumsticks are tender when pressed. Remove chicken to hot platter; skim all but 2 tbs. of basting fat out of pan and stir in shallots or scallions. Cook on stove, stirring for a moment and then add bouillon. Boil rapidly, scraping coagulated cooking juices into bouillon until liquid has reduced to a syrupy consistency. Pour over chicken and serve. Serves four.

TOTAL CALORIES PER PORTION: 280
CARB. CALORIES PER PORTION: 20

Artichokes and Shrimp Casserole à la Adlai

1 No. 2 can artichoke hearts *or* 1 pkg. frozen artichoke hearts cooked	1 tbs. worcestershire sauce
	Salt and pepper
	¼ c. good dry sherry wine
½ lb. medium-sized shrimp	¼ c. grated parmesan cheese
2 tbs. butter	1 c. cream sauce
¼ lb. fresh or canned mush- rooms	Dash of paprika

Drain can of whole artichokes and arrange in buttered baking dish. Spread the cooked shrimps over them. Sauté sliced mushrooms in butter for 6 minutes, and add them to baking dish. Add worcestershire sauce, salt, pepper and sherry to cream sauce, and pour contents of the baking dish. Sprinkle the top with parmesan cheese, dust with paprika and bake for 20 minutes in 375° oven. Cover dish with chopped parsley just before serving. Serves four.

TOTAL CALORIES PER PORTION: 340
CARB. CALORIES PER PORTION: 22

Chop Suey

1 lb. lean pork, cut in thin strips
2 tbs. cooking oil
½ c. sliced onions
1 c. celery, cut in thin strips
½ c. green pepper, cut in thin strips
1 ¼ c. water
1 bouillon cube

1 tbs. cornstarch
1 can (16 oz.) bean sprouts, drained
1 can (5 oz.) water chestnuts, drained and sliced
½ tsp. salt
2 tbs. soy sauce

Cook pork in hot oil until well seared, stirring. Add onions, celery and green pepper; cook 3 minutes. Add 1 cup of the water and the bouillon cube. Mix cornstarch with remaining ¼ cup water. Add to vegetable mixture; cook just until thick. Add bean sprouts, water chestnuts, salt and soy sauce; heat. Vegetables will be crisp. Serves four.

TOTAL CALORIES PER PORTION: 20
CARB. CALORIES PER PORTION: 14

Onion Gravy

1 envelope dry onion soup mix
1 tbs. unsifted flour

2 c. boiling water

Combine soup mix and flour. Stir to blend. Add water gradually, mixing well.

TOTAL CALORIES PER PORTION: 450
CARB. CALORIES PER PORTION: 30

Buffet Burgers

2 lb. ground chuck or round
¾ c. wheat germ
2 eggs
½ c. half and half
2 tbs. minced onion

2 tsp. worcestershire sauce
2 tsp. salt
¼ tsp. marjoram
¼ tsp. thyme

Combine all ingredients. Mix well. Shape into 8 patties, about 4 inches in diameter. Broil, fry or grill until done as desired, turning once. Serve plain or with cheese olive topping (recipe follows). Serves eight.

TOTAL CALORIES PER PORTION: 400

CARB. CALORIES PER PORTION: 22

Knockwurst and Sauerkraut

1 lb. knockwurst	2 tbs. brown pan drippings
2 lb. sauerkraut	from an oven roast *or*
1 sm. onion, chopped	2 tbs. butter
1 tbs. caraway seed	

Sauté onion until golden brown in pan drippings or butter. Add sauerkraut, caraway seed and about 1 cup of water. Cover and simmer about one hour. Place knockwurst on top of sauerkraut (adding small amount of water if necessary). Cover and continue to simmer for another 15 minutes. Serves four.

TOTAL CALORIES PER PORTION: 375

CARB. CALORIES PER PORTION: 22

Shrimp Newburg

1 lb. raw shrimp, shelled and deveined	3 egg yolks slightly beaten
	½ tsp. salt
4 tbs. butter or margerine	Dash pepper
1 c. light cream	2 tbs. sherry

If shrimp are large, cut into pieces. Melt butter in a skillet. Add shrimp and saute until shrimp are cooked (about 2 to 5 minutes), stirring frequently. Mix together egg yolks and cream. Heat in top part of double boiler over hot (not boiling) water, stirring constantly until mixture thickens. Add shrimp and continue cooking only until heated, being careful not to let the mixture boil. Add seasonings and sherry. Serves four.

TOTAL CALORIES PER PORTION: 285

CARB. CALORIES PER PORTION: 54

Wheat-Meat Loaf

1 lb. ground beef	1 tbs. worcestershire sauce
½ lb. ground pork	1 tbs. chopped onion
1 c. wheat germ	1 tsp. prepared mustard
¾ c. milk or tomato juice	½ tsp. salt
1 egg	

Combine all ingredients in large bowl, mixing well. Shape firmly into a round, flat loaf about 1 inch thick. Place in heavy 10-inch skillet or electric frypan. Cut almost through meat loaf with knife into desired number of pie-shaped servings. Prepare onion gravy (as in following recipe). Pour over meat. Cover and simmer for 30 minutes or until meat is done as desired. Serves six to eight.

TOTAL CALORIES PER PORTION: 80
CARB. CALORIES PER PORTION: 5

Cheese Olive Topping

1 c. shredded cheddar cheese	⅓ c. blue cheese, crumbled
¼ c. salad dressing	2 tbs. chopped stuffed olives
⅛ tsp. garlic powder	

Combine cheddar cheese, salad dressing and garlic powder. Mix well. Stir in blue cheese and olives.

TOTAL CALORIES PER PORTION: 310
CARB. CALORIES PER PORTION: 17

Swiss Omelet

½ c. milk	¼ lb. processed American
¼ c. wheat germ	cheese, shredded
4 eggs, separated	¼ lb. (½ c.) fully cooked,
½ tsp. salt	diced Canadian bacon
1 tbs. butter or margarine	

Combine milk and wheat germ. Set aside until ready to use. Beat egg whites until stiff but not dry. Beat egg yolks and salt until thick and lemon-colored. Fold yolks and wheat germ-milk mixture into beaten egg whites very carefully until mixture is well blended. Melt butter in 10-inch skillet with oven-proof handle. Pour egg mixture into pan, spreading gently until level. Cook uncovered over low heat until puffy and lightly browned on bottom and sides (about 10 minutes). Bake at 325° for 10 minutes or until a knife inserted in center comes out clean. Sprinkle cheese and bacon over omelet a few minutes before removing omelet from oven. Fold omelet slightly off center. Turn out onto warm platter. Serves three to four.

TOTAL CALORIES PER PORTION: 500
CARB. CALORIES PER PORTION: 20

Chicken in Cream With Chives

1 broiler-fryer, disjointed	Salt and pepper
¼ c. butter	½ c. minced chives
2 tbs. minced shallots or scallions	1¼ c. light cream
⅓ c. dry white wine	1 tbs. cornstarch

Sauté chicken pieces in butter until light golden brown; add the shallots or scallions and cook, stirring, until soft. Add the wine. Salt and pepper. Cover and simmer until chicken is tender, about 45 minutes. Meanwhile, combine 1 cup of cream and chives, mix the cornstarch with the remaining ¼ cup. When the chicken is done, place on serving dish, add the cornstarch mixture, then the chives and cream, stirring well. Cook until sauce thickens, then pour over chicken. Serves four.

TOTAL CALORIES PER PORTION: 330
CARB. CALORIES PER PORTION: 16

Salmon Loaf

1 can (1 lb.) salmon	¼ tsp. pepper
½ c. chopped celery	2 cups milk
¼ c. chopped onion	4 eggs, slightly beaten
⅛ c. butter or margarine	½ cup wheat germ
2 tbs. flour	2 tbs. chopped parsley
1 tsp. salt	1 tbs. lemon juice

Prepare salmon. Drain and save liquid; remove skin and bones. Sauté celery and onion in butter until onion is tender. Remove celery and onion and set aside. Blend flour, salt and pepper into melted butter until smooth. Add milk all at once. Cook over medium heat until mixture thickens, stirring constantly. Remove 1 cup of sauce for hot tartar sauce (recipe follows). Place in saucepan. Combine remaining sauce with salmon, salmon liquid, celery, onion and remaining ingredients. Mix well. Pour into greased, aluminum foil-lined 9 x 5 x 3 inch loaf pan. Bake at 350° for 45 minutes or until firm. Let stand in pan for 10 minutes. Turn out onto serving plate. Slice and serve with hot tartar sauce. Serves six.

TOTAL CALORIES PER PORTION: 80
CARB. CALORIES PER PORTION: 16

Hot Tartar Sauce

1 c. sauce (from salmon loaf recipe)	¼ c. pickle relish
¼ c. salad dressing	1 tbs. lemon juice

Measure all ingredients into saucepan. Mix well. Heat slowly over low heat, stirring frequently.

TOTAL CALORIES PER PORTION: 440
CARB. CALORIES PER PORTION: 33

Louisiana Steaks

6 pork shoulder steaks, cut ¾ inch thick	Louisiana sauce (recipe follows)
Salt and pepper	

Brown steaks on both sides in skillet. Pour off drippings. Season with salt and pepper. Prepare sauce and pour over steaks. Bake at 350° F. for 1 hour. Serves 6.

TOTAL CALORIES PER PORTION: 600
CARB. CALORIES PER PORTION: 37

Chicken Fricassee

1 stewing chicken 4 to 5 lb. cut up	1 medium onion
3 c. hot water	1 bay leaf
Parsley	2 tbs. flour
Salt	¼ c. milk
¼ tsp. white pepper	Dash of lemon juice
2 stalks celery	Paprika

Put chicken pieces in large, heavy kettle. Add the water, parsley, salt and next 4 ingredients. Bring to boil, cover and simmer 2 or 3 hours. (Cooking time depends on age and tenderness of chicken.) Remove chicken, strain broth and skim off fat. Return 2 cups broth to kettle. Blend flour and milk, stir gradually into broth and simmer a few minutes. Add chicken and heat gently. Season with salt and add lemon juice. Arrange chicken and gravy on platter. Sprinkle with chopped parsley and paprika. **Serves four.**

TOTAL CALORIES PER PORTION: 40
CARB. CALORIES PER PORTION: 30

Louisiana Sauce

¼ c. minced onion	1 tbs. butter or margarine
1 clove garlic, minced	1 tbs. flour
1½ tsp. chopped parsley	1½ c. tomato juice
1 can (4 oz.) sliced mushrooms (with liquid)	1 tsp. salt
¼ c. minced green pepper	½ tsp. sugar

Cook chopped vegetables in butter until they are lightly browned. Add flour and stir until smooth. Gradually add the tomato juice and seasonings. Cook, stirring, until thickened.

TOTAL CALORIES PER PORTION: 200
CARB. CALORIES PER PORTION: 20

Schinkenschoberl in Rindsuppe

(Ham-Egg Squares in Beef Broth)

1 tbs. butter or margarine	⅛ tsp. pepper
2 tbs. chopped onion	2 tbs. snipped parsley
⅓ c. diced boiled ham	¼ c. wheat germ
2 eggs separated	1 10½ oz. can condensed beef broth
¼ tsp. salt	

Start heating oven to 375° F. In hot butter or margarine, in small saucepan, sauté onion with ham till golden; set aside. In small bowl, with electric mixer at high speed, beat egg whites with salt untill stiff; fold in pepper, parsley, beaten egg yolks, wheat germ, ham mixture. Pour into well-greased 8" x 2" baking dish; bake 15 min.; cool; then cut into 1-inch squares. To serve: heat broth by label. Place a few ham and egg squares in each soup bowl, fill with broth. Serves four to six.

TOTAL CALORIES PER PORTION: 470
CARB. CALORIES PER PORTION: 35

Coq au Vin

4 whole chicken breasts (about 3 lb.)	1 ½ tsp. dried marjoram
2 strips bacon	1 bay leaf
1 lb. sm. fresh mushrooms	1 tsp. ground thyme
1 lb. sm. white onions	2 tbs. salt
3 carrots	⅛ tsp. black pepper
2 cloves garlic	1 tbs. meat-extract paste
2 medium onions	1½ c. dry red wine
1 tbs. salad oil	1 cup water
¼ c. snipped parsley	2 tbs. flour
	Salt and pepper

Day before serving: Split and skin chicken breasts. Cut bacon into ½ in. pieces. In a large dutch oven, fry bacon until almost crisp. Sauté a few chicken breasts at a time, until golden on all sides. Remove each piece as done. Meanwhile, wash mushrooms and trim, as necessary; cut any large mushrooms in half. Peel onions. Scrape carrots; cut into 1-inch slices. Mince garlic. Chop medium onions. In salad oil, in same dutch oven, saute mushrooms, white onions and carrots until onions begin to brown lightly; remove all. Saute garlic and chopped onions in remaining fat until onions are golden. Return chicken breasts to dutch oven and cover with sautéed vegetable mixture. Add parsley, marjoram, bay leaf, thyme, salt, pepper, meat-extract paste, wine and water. Cover, heat simmer gently for 20 minutes. Cool slightly; refrigerate, covered.

About 1 hour and 10 minutes before serving: Heat refrigerated mixture to a boil; then simmer, covered for 40 minutes or until chicken is tender and meat begins to come away from bones. Then mix enough water with flour to form a smooth, rather thin, paste. Remove chicken to a warm spot. Stirring constantly, add flour paste to chicken stock; simmer, stirring continually, until thickened and smooth. Add salt and pepper to taste. With slotted spoon, remove vegetables from gravy and circle around chicken. Spoon on some gravy; pass remaining gravy. Serves six.

TOTAL CALORIES PER PORTION: 660
CARB. CALORIES PER PORTION: 25

Chicken in Wine Sauce

One broiler-fryer (3 lb.) cut up   ⅛ tsp. cinnamon
¼ c. olive oil   ⅛ tsp. cloves
1 clove garlic, minced   1 c. dry white wine
2 tbs. minced onion   ¼ cup minced parsley
1 tsp. salt

Heat the oil and garlic in heavy skillet. Put in chicken; brown on all sides. Add onion, cooking until soft. Add salt, cinnamon, cloves and wine; cover and cook until chicken is tender. Remove chicken to platter; stir parsley in pan. Serves four.

TOTAL CALORIES PER PORTION: 300
CARB. CALORIES PER PORTION: 10

Seattle Salmon Steaks

6 salmon steaks, 1 in. thick   ¼ tsp. paprika
⅓ c. butter or margarine   1 tsp. worcestershire sauce
½ tsp. salt   2 tbs. grated onion

Place salmon steaks in greased shallow baking pan. Melt butter; add seasonings and worcestershire sauce; spread over salmon. Sprinkle 1 tsp. onion over each steak. Bake in moderate oven (350°) 25 to 30 minutes. Serves six.

TOTAL CALORIES PER PORTION: 250
CARB. CALORIES PER PORTION: 20

Brazilian Omelet con Carne

Sauce

1 c. ground leftover cooked beef   ½ tsp. salt
1 tbs. fat or salad oil   ¼ tsp. chili powder
1½ c. canned tomatoes   ½ green pepper, cut in strips

Omelet

6 egg yolks   Dash pepper
3 tbs. tomato juice   6 stiffly beaten egg whites
1 tsp. salt   3 tbs. fat or salad oil

Brown meat in 1 tbs. fat; add tomatoes, salt, chili powder, and green pepper; cook 10 minutes, stirring frequently. Beat egg yolks until light-colored and thick; add tomato juice and seasonings. Fold in whites. Heat 3 tbs. fat in skillet; pour in egg mixture; cover over very low heat until mixture puffs, about 8 minutes. Uncover, bake in slow oven (325°) 15 minutes, or brown under broiler. Fold. Pour souce over. Serves six.

TOTAL CALORIES PER PORTION: 157
CARB. CALORIES PER PORTION: 20

Broiled Seafood Cakes

12 oz. finely chopped cooked
  shrimp, lobster or crab
  meat
2 tbs. chopped parsley
1 tbs. chopped fresh dill

¼ tsp. curry
Salt and pepper
2 eggs
Milk

Mix sea food with herbs and seasonings. Break in eggs. Mix vigorously. Add enough milk to allow for shaping the mixture into cakes. Broil on both sides until well browned. Serves three to four.

TOTAL CALORIES PER PORTION: 300
CARB. CALORIES PER PORTION: 40

Seafood Casserole

1½ c. chopped celery
1 roast pimento
3 tsp. dehydrated onion
  flakes
4 tbs. fish stock or water

Ground ginger
1 can crab meat, flaked
1 can shrimp
¾ c. french dressing

Cook celery, pimento and dehydrated onion in fish stock or water. When most of the liquid has boiled away and vegetables are soft, season with ground ginger. Arrange in a casserole: a layer of vegetables, a layer of crab meat, a layer of vegetables, and a layer of shrimp. Top with french dressing and bake in moderate oven (350°) for half an hour. Serves four to five.

TOTAL CALORIES PER PORTION: 380
CARB. CALORIES PER PORTION: 28

Creme St. Jacques

1 lb. fresh bay or sea scallops
2 c. dry white wine
2 tbs. chopped shallots
4 sprigs parsley
3 tbs. butter

¼ tsp. cayenne pepper
6 coarsely chopped mushrooms
Salt and pepper
1 cup heavy cream
3 egg yolks, lightly beaten

If bay scallops are used, leave them whole. If sea scallops are used, cut in halves or quarters. Combine the scallops with the wine, shallots, parsley, butter, cayenne, mushrooms, salt and pepper. Bring to a boil and simmer 5 minutes. Strain and reserve both the liquid and the scallops. If desired the scallops may be chilled and mixed with mayonnaise and capers to make a first course. Return the liquid to the simmer. Combine the cream and egg yolks. Add to the liquid and stir rapidly with a whisk. Do not boil; cook slowly until soup is thickened slightly. Serve piping hot. Serves four to six.

TOTAL CALORIES PER PORTION: 300

CARB. CALORIES PER PORTION: 20

Swordfish Kabobs

2 lb. swordfish

1 4 oz. can button mushrooms, drained

2 tbs. lemon juice

½ c. french dressing

Cut fish into large chunks. Sprinkle with lemon juice. Marinate in french dressing. String on skewers alternating with mushrooms, and broil, turning once. Serves four.

TOTAL CALORIES PER PORTIONS 350

CARB. CALORIES PER PORTION: 30

Ham and Chicken Potage

½ c. diced cooked ham

2 tbs. chopped onion

2 tbs. butter

1 can condensed cream of chicken soup

½ soup can of milk

½ soup can of water

½ c. cooked, cut asparagus

Shredded milk-process cheese

Brown ham and onion in butter until tender. Blend in soup, milk, and water; add asparagus. Heat. Stir now and then. Do not boil. Garnish with cheese. Serves three.

TOTAL CALORIES PER PORTION: 370

CARB. CALORIES PER PORTION: 26

Chicken Tetrazzini

2 tbs. margarine

½ c. diced green pepper

½ lb. fresh mushrooms, sliced

1 clove garlic, crushed

½ c. sherry

1½ c. water

1 envelope chicken soup mix

1½ c. milk

1 tbs. cornstarch

3 c. cooked chicken chunks

1¼ c. grated parmesan cheese

¼ c. chopped parsley

Melt margarine in skillet. Add green pepper; cook over low heat 4 minutes, stirring frequently. Add mushrooms and garlic; cook until tender, stirring occasionally. Add sherry. Remove from heat. Bring water to a boil in saucepan. Add soup mix; cook gently 4 minutes. Blend in a little of the milk with the corn starch; stir in remaining milk. Stir into soup. Stirring constantly, bring to boil and boil 1 minute. Add chicken, 1 cup of cheese, parsley and green pepper-mushroom mixture. Divide into 6 individual baking dishes; sprinkle remaining cheese on top. Bake in hot oven for 10 minutes. Serves six.

TOTAL CALORIES PER PORTION: 410
CARB. CALORIES PER PORTION: 20

Hungarian Goulash

2 lb. veal cubes (1 inch)
2 tbs. shortening
1 can condensed tomato soup
½ c. sour cream

½ c. water
1 large clove garlic, minced
1 tsp. paprika
¼ tsp. salt

In large heavy pan, brown veal in shortening; pour off fat. Stir in remaining ingredients. Cover. Cook over low heat 1½ hours, or until meat is tender. Stir now and then. Serves four to six.

TOTAL CALORIES PER PORTION: 500
CARB. CALORIES PER PORTION: 30

Beef Chop Suey

1 lb. lean shoulder steak, cut into thin slices
2 tbs. cooking oil
1 c. sliced mushrooms
1 tbs. dehydrated onion
1½ c. water
1 beef bouillon cube

1½ tbs. soy sauce
⅛ tsp. pepper
1 c. thinly sliced celery
2 green peppers sliced in thin rings

Brown meat, mushrooms and onions in heavy iron skillet. Cook remaining ingredients in saucepan for 30 minutes. Add browned meat. Cover and simmer for a few minutes or until meat is tender. Serves four.

TOTAL CALORIES PER PORTION: 462
CARB. CALORIES PER PORTION: 18

Pot Roast

3 lb. pot roast of beef
1 tsp. salt
⅛ tsp. pepper
½ tsp. ground ginger
1 clove garlic, minced
1 carrot, cut up
¼ c. coarsely chopped parsley

½ c. water
½ c. tomato juice
1 onion, sliced
2 stalks celery, sliced
½ c. green beans
1 tomato, quartered

Combine salt, pepper, and ginger and rub mixture thoroughly into meat. Heat a heavy dutch oven and brown meat thoroughly on all sides over moderate heat. Add remaining ingredients (except tomato). Cover tightly and cook over very low heat about 3–4 hours or until meat is tender. Remove meat and let it cool slightly to make slicing easier. Add tomato and continue to cook about 5 minutes until tomato is softened. Serves four.

TOTAL CALORIES PER PORTION: 510
CARB. CALORIES PER PORTION: 32

Beef and Eggplant Casserole

1 lb. lean beef, cut into	Pepper
½-inch cubes	1 tsp. oregano
1 eggplant, peeled and sliced	½ c. tomato juice
2 green peppers, diced	½ c. water
Onion powder or flakes	1 tomato, sliced (optional)
Salt	

Brown meat well in heavy preheated pan. In a casserole, arrange layers of meat, eggplant, and peppers, seasoning each layer with onion, salt, pepper and oregano. Pour enough tomato juice and water over it to moisten it very well. Top with tomato. Cover and bake in 350° F. oven for 1 hour. Remove cover and bake 15 minutes more to brown top. Serves four.

TOTAL CALORIES PER PORTION: 476
CARB. CALORIES PER PORTION: 13

Pepper Steak

2 lb. shoulder steak	2 tbs. soy sauce
2 c. bouillon	1 tsp. salt
1 clove garlic	2 green peppers (cut up)

Slice steak into pieces ¼ inch thick and brown in large pre-heated iron pan over moderately high flame, stirring constantly, about 2 minutes. Add 2 cups bouillon, garlic, soy sauce and salt. Cover and cook 5 minutes on moderate flame. Stir in peppers and cook additional 2 minutes. Serves four.

TOTAL CALORIES PER PORTION: 490
CARB. CALORIES PER PORTION: 30

Barbecued Frankfurters-Sauerkraut

¼ c. chopped onion	¼ c. tomato sauce
½ c. chopped green pepper	½ tsp. worcestershire sauce
¼ c. chicken stock	1 tsp. prepared mustard
1½ lb. frankfurters, boiled, then	½ tsp. salt
gashed in places	1 can sauerkraut, drained

Cook onion and green pepper until tender in saucepan, with chicken stock. Add frankfurters and brown slightly. Combine tomato sauce, worcestershire sauce, mustard and salt. Add to farnkfurters. Cook slowly about 10 minutes. Spoon sauerkraut into a two-quart casserole. Arrange franks on sauerkraut and pour sauce over all. Cover tightly and bake in a 350° F. oven for 20 minutes. Serves six.

TOTAL CALORIES PER PORTION: 463
CARB. CALORIES PER PORTION: 22

Sauerbraten

1 c. vinegar
1 c. water
½ tsp. salt
5 peppercorns
⅛ tsp. cloves

3 bay leaves
2 onions, chopped
2 carrots, sliced
3 lb. piece beef (chuck or top round)

Bring first 8 ingredients to a boil to make a marinade. Place meat in a bowl. Pour marinade over it. Refrigerate 2–3 days, turning the meat frequently. Drain meat, reserving marinade. Brown meat over low heat in very hot dutch oven. Add marinade. Cover and cook over low heat for 3 hours or until meat is tender. Serves six.

TOTAL CALORIES PER PORTION: 300
CARB. CALORIES PER PORTION: 17

Hamburger Meal in One Dish

1½ lb. lean chopped meat
½ c. finely chopped celery
1 sm. onion, chopped
1 c. mushrooms, chopped
1 c. tomato juice

1 c. water
Salt and pepper
1 pkg. frozen green beans, cooked and drained

Brown meat, celery and onion in heavy skillet, stirring often. Transfer to casserole, draining off all fat. Add mushrooms, tomato juice, salt and pepper, and green beans. Bake at 350° F. for 30 minutes. Serves four.

TOTAL CALORIES PER PORTION: 242
CARB. CALORIES PER PORTION: 26

Stuffed Peppers

1 lb. lean ground beef
¼ tsp. salt
⅛ tsp. pepper
Onion powder to taste
1 clove garlic, pressed
½ lb. mushrooms, cooked and chopped

1 tsp. crushed leaf sage
1½ tbs. chopped parsley
4 tbs. water
6 medium green peppers
2 pkg. bouillon dissolved in 1 c. hot water

Preheat oven to 350° F. Mix chopped meat with salt, pepper, onion, garlic, mushrooms, leaf sage and parsley. Moisten slightly with water. Divide into 6 equal parts. Wash and remove tops of 6 peppers. Discard seeds. Soften by dropping them in boiling water for 5 minutes. Fill cavities with ground-meat mixture. Place in baking dish, pour in bouillon and bake until peppers are tender, about 25 minutes. Serves six.

TOTAL CALORIES PER PORTION: 330

CARB. CALORIES PER PORTION: 55

Veal and Kidney Shish-Kebab

1 lb. veal kidneys	½ tsp. salt
1 lb. veal for stewing	½ tsp. pepper
Meat tenderizer	½ tsp. garlic powder
2 large green peppers	½ tsp. onion powder
4 medium onions	¾ c. soy sauce

Wash and clean kidneys thoroughly. Cut in half lengthwise. Soak cleaned kidneys in salted water holding 2 tbs. vinegar for 30 minutes. While kidneys are soaking sprinkle meat tenderizer on veal cubes following directions on bottle. Cut green peppers into 2 inch cubes. Peel and cut onions into quarters. Remove kidneys from water and rinse with cold water. Place all ingredients in bowl and cover with remaining spices and soy sauce. Marinate overnight. Alternate meat and vegetables on skewers. Broil until brown and tender, turning and basting with remaining marinade. Serves four.

TOTAL CALORIES PER PORTION: 300

CARB. CALORIES PER PORTION: 30

Chicken Cacciatora

2 lb. boneless chicken breasts, cut into 8 pieces	Salt and pepper
	¼ tsp. dried thyme
2 sm. green peppers	6 sprigs parsley
1 clove garlic	1½ c. sliced mushrooms
2 tbs. finely chopped pimiento	2 c. stewed tomatoes
1 bay leaf	

Combine all ingredients in saucepan. Simmer 30 minutes. Uncover and continue cooking until sauce is reduced to desired consistency. Serves four.

TOTAL CALORIES PER PORTION: 600

CARB. CALORIES PER PORTION: 0

Roast Squab

Wash and dry 4 squabs, using paper towels. Rub inside with salt and pepper. Rub with a small amount of salad oil. Place in roasting pan, side by side, and bake uncovered in moderate oven (350°) about 45 to 60 minutes or until tender. Serves four.

TOTAL CALORIES PER PORTION: 125

CARB. CALORIES PER PORTION: 5

Shirred Eggs

Place 1 tbs. cream in each of 4 greased custard cups. Break an egg into each; sprinkle with salt and pepper, and bake in slow oven (325°) till eggs are firm, about 20 minutes. Variations may be obtained by adding either ¼ c. chopped cooked spinach, or a slice of bacon, or canned pimientos to the custard cup before breaking the egg into it. Serves four.

VEGETABLES

TOTAL CALORIES PER PORTION: 80
CARB. CALORIES PER PORTION: 30

Eggplant Fresno

1½ tsp. butter or margarine
1 med. onion, thinly sliced
¼ med. green pepper, chopped
1 med. eggplant, peeled and cut into ¾ in. cubes

1 1-lb can tomatoes
½ tsp. salt
1 tsp. sugar

In butter or margarine, in a medium skillet or saucepan with a tight-fitting cover, saute onion and green pepper until onion is golden. Add eggplant cubes, tomatoes, salt and sugar; cover; simmer 10 minutes or until eggplant is just tender. Serves six.

TOTAL CALORIES PER PORTION: 50
CARB. CALORIES PER PORTION: 25

Green Beans Sorrento

1 strip bacon
¼ c. finely chopped onion
1 clove garlic, minced
2 tbs. chopped green pepper
1 med. tomato, chopped

2 pkg. frozen French-style green beans, partly thawed
½ tsp. oregano
1¼ tsp. salt
⅛ tsp. black pepper
¼ c. water

Cut bacon into small pieces. In a medium skillet with a tight-fitting cover, sauté bacon until lightly browned. Add onion, garlic and green pepper; saute until golden. Stir in tomato pieces, green beans, oregano, salt, pepper and water; cover; simmer 13 minutes or until green beans are tender-crisp. Serves six.

SALADS

TOTAL CALORIES PER PORTION: 160
CARB. CALORIES PER PORTION: 40

Greek Salad

4 cucumbers
2 bu. radishes
1 c. pitted ripe olives
8 oz. feta or muenster cheese

½ c. bottled oil and vinegar dressing
1 bu. scallions, sliced

One hour ahead: Halve cucumbers lengthwise; seed, quarter length-wise; cut crosswise, in thirds. Toss with sliced radishes, olives and scallions. Chill. To serve—toss with dressing and cheese cut in strips. Serves eight.

TOTAL CALORIES PER PORTION: 60

CARB. CALORIES PER PORTION: 16

Egg and Onion Sambal

1 lg. sweet onion, thinly sliced	⅓ c. lemon juice
1 med. cucumber, thinly sliced	⅓ c. water
1 lg. green pepper sliced ⅛ in. thick	½ tsp. sugar
	1 tsp. salt
3 hard boiled eggs, halved	¼ tsp. pepper

In a bowl combine onion, cucumber and green pepper. Combine lemon juice, water, sugar, salt and pepper. Pour over vegetables. Toss together thoroughly. Chill for several hours. Just before serving, toss again. Garnish with hard-boiled eggs. Serves four to six.

TOTAL CALORIES PER PORTION: 137

CARB. CALORIES PER PORTION: 44

Pineapple Cheese Salad

1 pkg. (3 oz.) cream cheese, softened	6 slices canned low-calorie pineapple
3 tbs. wheat germ	6 lettuce leaves
1 tbs. juice from canned pine-apple	Salad dressing, if desired

Combine cream cheese, wheat germ and juice. Shape into 1-inch balls. Roll in additional wheat germ, if desired. Arrange pineapple slice on lettuce leaf. Top with cheese ball. Serve with dressing, if desired. Serves six.

TOTAL CALORIES PER PORTION: 270

CARB. CALORIES PER PORTION: 22

Christina's Cole Slaw

1 medium head cabbage, shred-ded	¼ c. light cream or milk
4 carrots, scraped and grated	6 tbs. finely minced onion
1 c. mayonnaise	Salt and freshly ground pepper to taste

Combine cabbage and carrots in large salad bowl and refrigerate. Mix together mayonnaise, cream or milk and onion. Let stand in refrigerator at least 20 minutes. Pour dressing over vegetables, toss lightly and season to taste. Serve immediately or keep refrigerated until ready to serve. Serves eight.

TOTAL CALORIES PER PORTION: 220
CARB. CALORIES PER PORTION: 20

Asparagus Vinaigrette

2 lb. fresh asparagus, cooked	Dash pepper
3 tbs. cider vinegar	½ tsp. sugar
¼ c. salad oil	1 hard-cooked egg, chopped
2 tbs. olive oil	2 sweet pickles, chopped
2 tsp. salt	

Arrange cooked asparagus spears in shallow baking dish. In jar with tight lid, combine vinegar, oils, salt, pepper, and sugar; shake to combine. Pour dressing over asparagus. Refrigerate at least 1 hour, turning spears several times. Arrange asparagus on a platter, sprinkle with chopped egg and pickle. Serves six.

TOTAL CALORIES PER PORTION: 45
CARB. CALORIES PER PORTION: 40

Cucumbers Vinaigrette

¼ c. Italian-style dressing	¼ tsp. crushed garlic
2 tbs. lemon juice	2 cucumbers, quartered and sliced ¼ in. thick
1 tbs. chopped capers	
1 tsp. worcestershire sauce	8 lettuce leaves

Combine dressing, lemon juice, capers, worcestershire and garlic; mix well. Pour over cucumbers in shallow dish; refrigerate covered about one hour. With slotted spoon, lift and drain cucumbers; sprinkle dressing over lettuce. Arrange lettuce on 8 salad plates; top with cucumbers. Serves eight.

TOTAL CALORIES PER PORTION: 290
CARB. CALORIES PER PORTION: 35

Mardi Gras Cole Slaw

3 c. finely shredded green cabbage	3 tsp. vinegar
3 c. finely shredded red cabbage	1 tsp. sugar
	⅔ c. shredded carrots
2 tsp. salt	⅔ c. sliced ripe olives
1¼ c. mayonnaise	½ c. chopped green pepper

Cover cabbage with cold water together with ½ tsp. salt; let soak for 1 hour. Drain. Combine mayonnaise, vinegar, sugar and remaining salt in large bowl. Add cabbage, carrot, olives and green pepper; toss lightly until vegetables are well coated. Refrigerate, covered for several hours. Serves six–eight.

TOTAL CALORIES PER PORTION: 260

CARB. CALORIES PER PORTION: 20

Make-A-Meal Salad Bowl

1 clove garlic, cut in half

½ head lettuce, broken into 1½ in. chunks

2 tbs. chopped green pepper

½ c. sliced celery

½ c. thinly sliced raw cauliflowerets

1 c. cooked asparagus tips

1 hard-cooked egg, cut in 8ths

½ lb. baked ham or salami, cut Julienne style

½ c. french dressing

Rub inside of salad bowl with cut surface of garlic clove, then discard garlic. Combine remaining ingredients in order given; add dressing, toss lightly until each piece of salad is coated with dressing. Six to eight servings.

TOTAL CALORIES PER PORTION: 250

CARB. CALORIES PER PORTION: 43

Shrimp salad

1 lb. fresh cooked shrimp

2 c. sliced celery

¼ tsp. salt

1 tsp. sugar

½ tsp. dry mustard

⅛ tsp. paprika

2 tsp. horseradish

½ c. salad oil

2 tbs. vinegar

Prepare shrimp and celery. Mix dry ingredients together; add horseradish, salad oil and vinegar. Blend well. Pour over shrimp and chill in refrigerator 2 hours. Add celery. Serve on lettuce. Serves four–five.

TOTAL CALORIES PER PORTION: 12

CARB. CALORIES PER PORTION: 10

Perfection Salad

1 tbs. unflavored gelatin

½ c. cold water

1 c. sauerkraut juice, lemon juice and water combined

1 c. canned sauerkraut, drained

½ c. diced celery

1 tbs. grated onion

1 diced pimiento or 2 tbs. diced green or red pepper)

Sprinkle gelatin into small saucepan holding the cold water. Place over low heat and stir to dissolve gelatin. Add juice and water mixture; Chill to let thicken slightly. Cut up drained sauerkraut into small pieces. Add celery, grated onion, pimiento (or pepper). Combine with gelatin mixture, turn into small mold and chill several hours until firm. Unmold. Serve plain or with french dressing to which you add about 1 tsp. of horseradish sauce. Garnish with cucumber slices. Serves four–six.

TOTAL CALORIES PER PORTION: 275
CARB. CALORIES PER PORTION: 25

Plantation Tomato Salad

3 medium tomatoes, peeled, sliced

1 onion, peeled, cut into rings

Salad greens

⅓ c. french dressing

¾ tsp. celery seed

¼ c. pickle relish

6 slices crisp-cooked bacon, crumbled

3 hard-cooked eggs, quartered

Arrange tomato slices alternately with onion rings on salad greens. Combine dressing, celery seed and pickle relish; pour over tomatoes and onions. Sprinkle bacon on top. Garnish with egg sections. Serves six.

TOTAL CALORIES PER PORTION: 6
CARB. CALORIES PER PORTION: 3

"Roast Peanuts" (Mushrooms)

Canned button mushrooms
Salt

Drain all liquid from can. Spread mushrooms evenly on cookie tin or aluminum foil tray. Sprinkle generously with salt. Bake in slow oven, 250° F. about 1 hour, or until mushrooms are brown and completely dry. These taste very much like peanuts and can be eaten as a snack with no added weight penalty.

DESSERTS

TOTAL CALORIES PER PORTION: 155
CARB. CALORIES PER PORTION: 125

Zabaglione

5 egg yolks

4 tbs. granulated sugar

8 tbs. sweet marsala wine

Combine egg yolks, sugar and wine in the top of a large double boiler. Beat continuously for 7–8 minutes over hot, but not boiling, water. As you beat, the mixture will swell and, in the end, almost completely fill the top of the double boiler. It will be lukewarm, light-colored and thick and creamy in texture. Serve immediately in champagne glasses or stemmed drinking glasses. Serves four.

TOTAL CALORIES PER PORTION: 4
CARB. CALORIES PER PORTION: 3

Coffee Whip

1 envelope unflavored gelatin

¼ c. cold water

1½ c. hot strong coffee

½ tsp. sugar

½ tsp. vanilla

Dash of salt

Sprinkle gelatin on cold water to soften. Dissolve in hot coffee. Add remaining ingredients. Chill in mixing bowl until syrupy. Beat with rotary beater until mixture is almost double in volume. Spoon into 6 sherbert glasses. Chill until firm. Serves six.

TOTAL CALORIES PER PORTION: 160
CARB. CALORIES PER PORTION: 24

Cheese Pie

18 oz. cottage cheese
½ tsp. nutmeg
¼ tsp. cinnamon
½ tsp. rum flavoring
½ tsp. vanilla
½ tsp. sugar
2 eggs, separated

Combine all ingredients except egg whites in bowl of electric mixer. Beat at high speed until smooth. Do not underbeat. Fold in stiffly beaten egg whites. Place in 7-inch pie pan. Set on bottom shelf of broiler rack. Broil 8 minutes or until top is golden brown. Serve hot or cold and garnish with strawberries, if desired. Serves four.

TOTAL CALORIES PER PORTION: 28
CARB. CALORIES PER PORTION: 20

Lemon Gelatin

1 envelope unflavored gelatin
¾ c. cold water
Dash of salt
1 tsp. sugar
⅓ c. lemon or lime juice

Sprinkle gelatin over cold water in saucepan. Heat over low flame, stirring constantly. Add a dash of salt, sugar, and lemon or lime juice. Mix by stirring. Pour into individual wet molds and chill until firm. Serve with whipped cream if desired. Serves six.

TOTAL CALORIES PER PORTION: 23
CARB. CALORIES PER PORTION: 18

Strawberry Delight

1 envelope unflavored gelatin
¼ c. cold water
1½ c. strawberries
1 tsp. sugar
1 tbs. lemon juice
⅛ tsp. salt
¼ c. nonfat dry milk
¼ c. ice water

Soften gelatin in cold water; dissolve over boiling water. Mash strawberries; add sugar, lemon juice, and salt. Blend in softened gelatin; chill until mixture begins to thicken. Combine dry milk and ice water; beat on high speed of mixer until stiff; fold into gelatin. Spoon into a wet 1-quart mold. Chill. Serves four to six.

TOTAL CALORIES PER PORTION: 10
CARB. CALORIES PER PORTION: 6

Maple Bavarian Cream

1 envelope unflavored gelatin
2 c. water
2 tsp. instant coffee

1 tsp. sugar
1 sm. capful maple flavor
1 tsp. nonfat dry milk

Soften gelatin in ½ cup cold water. Bring 1½ cups water to boil. Add coffee, sugar, maple flavor and gelatin mixture. Mix well and chill. When it is jelled, put through blender with dry milk for 10–15 seconds. Refrigerate. This mixture will jell in about ½ hour in refrigerator after blending. Serves four to six.

TOTAL CALORIES PER PORTION: 75
CARB. CALORIES PER PORTION: 12

Spanish Cream Sponge

2 eggs, separated
2 c. milk
1 tbs. unflavored gelatin

1 tsp. sugar
Dash of salt
1 tsp. vanilla

In top of double boiler, mix lightly egg yolks, milk, gelatin, sugar, salt and vanilla. Cook over hot water for a few minutes until mixture coats the spoon, stirring constantly. Remove from heat. Whip egg whites until stiff and fold into hot mixture. Pour into 6 custard cups or one large gelatin mold and chill until set. Serves six.

TOTAL CALORIES PER PORTION: (Trace) Very little
CARB. CALORIES PER PORTION: (Trace) Very little

Soda Gelatin

1 bottle any flavor lo-cal soda
1 pkg. unflavored gelatin

Pour all but ¼ cup soda into a pot and heat to boiling. Combine the ¼ cup of soda and gelatin and add boiled soda. Pour into serving dishes and chill until set. Serves four.

Appendix II

Table of Protein, Fat and Carbohydrate Content of Popular Beverages and Foods by Calories

Alcohols	Total Calories		

Only total calories of alcoholic beverage servings are shown. Whiskey and dry wines have little or no carbohydrate content.

Absinthe, cocktail glass	49	Chartreuse 1 oz.	95
Ale, 1 glass	144	Creme de Cocao 1 oz.	75
Anisette, 1 oz.	75	Creme de Menthe 1 oz.	95
Bacardi cocktail, 1 oz.	60	Curacao 1 oz.	70
Beer, American 1 c.	115	Dacquiri cocktails 2 oz.	100
Beer, imported 1 c.	127	Dry wine, burgundy,	
Benedictine cocktail glass	80	chablis, claret, etc., ½ c.	75
Bitters, Angostura 1 tsp.	10	Gin 1 oz.	60
Brandy, apple or cognac 1		Gin fizz 2 oz.	60
oz.	70	Gin highball 3 oz.	90
Brandy, cherry 1 oz.	75	Gin rickey 3 oz.	60
Brandy fizz 1 oz.	75	Madiera wine ½ c.	130
Brandy flip 2 oz.	147	Malaga wine ½ c.	174
California red wine ½ c.	71	Manhattan cocktail 2 oz.	150
California white wine ½ c.	90	Martini cocktail 2 oz.	60
Camille cocktail ½ c.	239	Mint julep 4 oz.	140
Catawba wine ½ c.	121	Old-Fashioned cocktail 2 oz.	125
Champagne, dry ½ c.	85	Port wine, domestic ½ c.	173
Champagne, sweet ½ c.	117	Port wine, imported ½ c.	155

Alcohols   Calories

Alcohols		Calories	
Rum, Bacardi 2 oz.	120	Tom Collins ½ c.	118
Rum, Jamaica 1 oz.	123	Vermouth, dry 1 oz.	60
Sherry, California ½ c.	144	Vermouth, sweet 1 oz.	90
Sherry, dry imported ½ c.	128	Whiskey, bourbon, rye,	
Sherry flip ½ c.	193	blends etc. 1 oz.	70
Tokay, sweet wine ½ c.	123	Whiskey, scotch 1 oz.	60
Tom and Jerry 1 c.	266		

Beverages	Protein	Fat	Carbo-hydrate	Total Calories
Apple juice 1 c.	1		100	101
Blueberry juice 1 c.	1		110	111
Blackberry juice 1 c.	2		64	66
Chocolate, hot 1 c.	41	144	124	309
Cider 1 c.	1		100	101
Cocoa 1 c.	40	99	96	235
Coffee (Black)	—	—	—	—
Currant juice, black 1 c.	4		112	116
Currant juice, red 1 c.	2		81	83
Eggnog 1 c.	44	99	72	215
Fruit punch 1 c.	4	2	48	54
Ginger ale 1 c.			128	128
Grape juice 1 c.	3	2	80	85
Grapefruit juice, fresh 1 c.	3	2	80	85
Grapefruit juice 1 c. sweet	3	2	128	133
Grapefruit juice 1 c. unsweetened	3	2	88	93
Lemonade, plain 1 c.			82	82
Limeade 1 c.			84	84
Loganberry juice 1 c.	5		80	85
Orange juice 1 c.			80	80
Ovaltine 1 c.	24	61	56	144
Peach juice 1 c.	2		104	106
Pineapple juice 1 c.	2	2	104	108
Postum 1 c.	2		16	18
Prune juice 1 c.	3		155	158
Raspberry juice, black 1 c.	2		84	86
Raspberry juice, red 1 c.	3		68	71

Beverages	Protein	Fat	Carbo-hydrate	Calories
Root beer 1 c.	3		64	67
Sauerkraut juice 1 c.			1	1
Strawberry juice 1 c.	2		41	43
Tea (no sugar or cream)	—	—	—	—
Tomato juice 1 c.	8	4	36	48

Bread, Cereals & Crackers	Protein	Fat	Carbo-hydrate	Calories
Baking powder biscuit 1 2" x 2" diam.	12	45	72	129
Barley, pearl ½ c.	4	2	52	58
Bisquick 1 c.	52	126	316	494
Boston brown bread 3 sl. 3" diam.	20	18	160	198
Bran, wheat prepared ¼ c.	12	6	44	62
Bread, cracked wheat 1 sl. 4" x 4" x ½"	8	4	52	64
Bread, french 4½" x 3½" x 1"	12	3	60	75
Bread, gluten 1 sl. 4" x 4" x ⅜"	8	5	48	61
Bread, graham 1 sl. 4" x 4" x ⅜"	8	5	48	61
Bread nut 1 sl. 1" thick	24	18	108	150
Bread, pumpernickel 1 sl. 3¼" x 4" x ½"	12	5	80	97
Bread, raisin 1 sl. 4" x 4" x ½"	12	4	64	80
Bread, rye 1 sl. 3½" x 4" x ½"	12	4	64	80
Bread, wheat fortified, milk 1 sl.	8	5	52	65
Bread, white milk 1 sl. 4" x 4" x ½"	8	4	48	60
Bread, whole wheat 1 sl. 4" x 4" x ½"	12	2	48	62
Bun, cinnamon 1	12	18	76	106
Bun, currant 1	8	18	68	94
Butter crackers 2	4	9	28	41

Bread, Cereals & Crackers	*Protein*	*Fat*	*Carbo-hydrate*	*Calories*
Crackers, animal or alphabet ½ c.	12	45	160	217
Crackers, arrowroot 1	4	9	32	45
Crackers, cheese Ritz 4–5	8	36	40	84
Crackers, cheese sandwich 3″ or 2″ sq.	8	9	24	41
Crackers, Ritz 4–5	4	45	40	89
Crackers, Triscuit 2	4		32	36
Crackers, Uneeda 2	4	9	44	57
Crackers, whole wheat 2	4		16	20
Coffee cake 3″ x 2″ x 2½″	12	45	76	133
Cornflakes 1 c.	8	2	72	82
Corn bread 2″ x 4″ x 2½″	52	135	348	535
Cream of wheat 3 tbs. uncooked	12		80	92
Croutons, fried 18 of ½″ cube	8	63	44	115
Croutons, toasted 21–23 of ½″ cube	8		52	60
Farina ½ c.	8		56	64
Graham crackers 1 of 2¼″ x 2 ¾″	3	9	28	40
Grapenuts ⅓ c.	16		104	120
Griddle cakes 2 of 4½″ diam.	32	54	140	226
Hominy, yellow ½ c.	8		60	68
Macaroni ½ c.	16		99	115
Malt ⅓ c.	24	6	160	190
Muffins, blueberry 2 of 2″ diam.	8	18	72	98
Muffins, bran 1 of 2″ diam.	16	36	68	120
Muffins, cornmeal 1 of 2¾″ diam.	12	36	88	136
Muffins, English 1 large	24	72	184	280
Muffins, one egg 1 of 2¾″ diam.	20	27	64	111
Muffins, graham 1 of 2¾″ diam.	16	18	92	126

Bread, Cereals & Crackers	Protein	Fat	Carbo-hydrate	Calories
Muffins, soybean 2 of 2″ diam.	32	108	28	168
Noodles, egg uncooked ¼ c.	12	18	84	114
Oysters, crackers 10	4	9	28	41
Peanut butter crackers	12	45	60	117
Pilot crackers 1	12	9	76	97
Popcorn, popped 1 c.	8	4	52	64
Popovers 1 of 3″ x 2¾″	16	27	56	99
Pretzellettes 14–16	12	9	120	141
Pretzels 3 large	12	9	120	141
Pumpernickel bread 1 sl. 3½″ x 4″ x ½″	12	5	80	97
Rolls, French 1	12	9	88	109
Rolled oats uncooked 4 tbs.	16	18	76	110
Rolled oats ½ c.	12	9	52	73
Rolls, Parkerhouse 1	8	3	44	55
Rice, puffed 1 c.	4		52	56
Rice, white ⅔ c.	8		92	100
Rice, wild ½ c.	20		100	120
Roman meal ½ c.	20	9	96	125
Rye bread 1 sl. 3½″ x 4″ x ½″	12	4	64	80
Rye Krisp 1 wafer 1⅞″ x 3⅝″	4		20	24
Saltines 1 double	4	7	20	31
Spaghetti, plain cooked ½ c.	16		76	92
Tapioca ⅛ c.			56	56
Waffles, plain 1 of 6″ diam.	36	90	128	254
Wheat germ 2 tbs.	20	18	40	78
Wheat, puffed 1 c.	8		44	52
Wheat shredded 1 biscuit	12		88	100
Wheat toasted 1 c.	8		64	72

Cakes, Pies, Puddings, Ice Creams & Cookies	Protein	Fat	Carbo-hydrate	Calories
Angelfood cake 3″ arc 2″ x 2″	16	9	104	129
Apple pie 4½″ x 4½ x 1″	16	117	228	361
Applesauce cake 1″ x 1″ x 3½″	8	9	80	97

Cakes, Pies, Puddings, Ice Creams & Cookies	*Protein*	*Fat*	*Carbo-hydrate*	*Calories*
Apple snow pudding ¾ c.			88	88
Apple tapioca ½ c.			220	220
Apricot chiffon pie 4″ x 4½″ x 2″	16	117	132	265
Apricot ice ½ c.	16	27	192	235
Avocado ice cream ½ c.	16	207	72	295
Bavarian cream pudding ½ c.	12	81	60	153
Black or blueberry pie 4½″ arc	12	117	240	369
Boston cream pie 3″ arc	12	90	132	234
Bread pudding ½ c.	28	63	96	187
Brownies 2 of 2¾″ diam.	8	36	80	124
Butter cake 2½″ x 3″ x 1″	12	63	116	191
Butterscotch pie 3″ x 4½″ x 2″	20	117	140	277
Butterscotch sundae ½ c.	16	90	112	218
Cake, plain 2″ x 1″ x 2″	12	27	124	163
Cake, pound 2″ x 5″ x ½″	8	72	72	152
Caramel nut sundae ½ c.	12	81	124	217
Caramel pudding ½ c.	12	63	108	183
Carrot pudding 1⅛″ x 4″ diam.	8	63	92	163
Chocolate cake 1¼″ x 1½″ x 3″	20	114	164	298
Chocolate chiffon pie 3″ arc by 4½″ x 1″	32	162	180	374
Chocolate cookies 2 of 2¼″ diam.	12	90	60	162
Chocolate ice cream ½ c.	12	127	88	227
Chocolate nut sundae ½ c.	12	117	136	265
Chocolate pie 3″ x 4½″ x 2″ arc	20	81	120	221
Chocolate pudding ½ c.	28	99	104	231
Chocolate soufflé ½ c.	20	162	84	266
Chocolate wafers 3 of 3″ diam.	8	27	76	111

Cakes, Pies, Puddings, Ice Creams & Cookies	Protein	Fat	Carbo-hydrate	Calories
Cocoanut cake 1¼″ x 1½″ x 3″	15	36	116	167
Cocoanut cream pie 3½″ arc	20	90	160	270
Coffee chiffon pie 4″ x 4½″ x 2″ arc	20	81	100	201
Corn pudding ½ c.	8	27	144	179
Cream puff 1	20	81	100	201
Cranberry pie 3″ arc	8	81	176	165
Custard ice cream ½ c.	16	81	72	169
Custard Pie 4½″ arc	28	99	80	207
Custard pudding 1 custard c.	20	45	36	101
Date bars 1 3″ x 1½″ diam.	8	27	68	103
Date torte pudding 4″ x 2″ x 3″	16	126	256	398
Devil's food cake 2″ x 2″ x 1¾″	20	60	68	148
Doughnuts 1 large	12	99	104	215
Fig newtons 1	4		76	80
Fruit cake 2″ x 2″ x ¼″	8	27	60	95
Fudge nut sundae ½ c.	20	117	140	277
Fig, steamed pudding 2¼″ x ¼″	12	45	100	157
Fudge wafers 1 of 2½″ x 1½ x 1″	4	36	32	72
Gelatin dessert powder 1 box	40		352	392
Gingerbread 1″ x 2″ x 2″	4	36	68	108
Gingersnaps 2 of 3″ diam.	8	27	92	127
Grapenut pudding 1 custard c.	16	36	100	152
Hermits 2 of 2″ diam.	8	27	64	99
Icebox cookies 2-3 of 2″ diam.	8	36	56	100
One egg cake 2″ x 2″ x 1″	8	27	72	107
Orange cup cake 1 of 2½″ x 1¾″	12	54	116	182

Cakes, Pies, Puddings, Ice Creams & Cookies	Protein	Fat	Carbo-hydrate	Calories
Plain ice cream ½ c.	16	117	80	213
Jello ½ c.	12		100	112
Jello solution ½ c.	12		80	92
Jellyroll cake ½ sl. of 3¼″ diam.	16	27	140	183
Junket, choc. ½ c.	12	45	356	413
Junket powder, plain ½ c.			396	396
Lady Baltimore cake 4″ x 2″ x ¾″	4	45	96	145
Ladyfingers 2	8	6	40	54
Lemon chiffon pudding 4″ x 4″ x 3″	24	90	160	274
Lemon ice cream ½ c.			116	116
Lemon pie 4″ arc	12	98	152	262
Lorna Doone cookies 6 of 1¾″ diam.	12	99	132	243
Macaroons, cocoanut 2 of 1½″ diam.	8	45	40	93
Macaroons, bran 2 of 1¾″ diam.	8	18	72	98
Maple nut sundae ½ c.	16	108	116	240
Marguerites 2	12	45	52	109
Marshallow cookies 3 of 1″ diam.	16	72	136	224
Marshallow pudding 3½″ x 3″ x 1¾″	60	288	276	624
Milk sherbert ½ c.	8	27	100	135
Mince pie 4″ arc	32	99	196	327
Molasses cookies 2 of 3″ diam.	4	36	60	100
Nabisco cookies 4		18	28	46
Nut loaf cake 2″ x 2″ x 1″	8	63	68	139
Oatmeal cookies 1 of 3″ diam.	8	27	48	83
Oatmeal wafers 2 of 1½″ x 1″	4	18	40	62
Orange ice ½ c.			108	108

Cakes, Pies, Puddings, Ice Creams & Cookies	Protein	Fat	Carbo-hydrate	Calories
Orange thins, cookies 2 of 2¾" diam.	4	27	72	103
Oriental tea cookies 2	4	4	32	40
Pastry shell 8"	28	270	168	466
Pineapple nut sundae ½ c.	12	72	152	236
Plum pudding 4" diam. by 1"	8	18	88	114
Popsicle 1 ⅛"	25	81	100	206
Prune soufflé ½ c.	12		96	108
Peanut cookies 2 of 2" diam.	16	72	64	152
Prune pie 3½" arc	12	135	248	395
Pumpkin pie 4" arc	20	56	164	240
Raisin Pie 3" arc	20	117	256	393
Rice pudding with raisins	12	9	124	155
Rhubarb pie 4½" arc	16	81	212	309
Spice cake 2" x 2" x 1"	8	72	108	188
Sponge cake 1" x 2½" x 1¾"	16	27	108	151
Squash pie 4½ arc	16	63	116	195
Strawberry shortcake 1 large biscuit	20	99	136	255
Suet pudding 2 ¾" x ⅞"	20	45	132	197
Tamale pie 1 c.	148	144	92	384
Tapioca pudding 6 tbs.	16	27	88	131
Sandwich cookies 1–3	8	63	96	167
Sour cream cookies 2 of 2¼" diam.	8	27	72	107
Sugar cookies 2 of 3¼" diam.	4	72	88	164
Toast, cinnamon 1 sl. 4" x 4" x 1"	20	63	116	199
Toast, creamed 1 sl. 5 tbs. sauce	24	63	88	175
Toast, french 1 sl. 4" x 4" x ⅝"	20	63	84	167
Toast, melba 1 sl. 4" x 4" x ¼"	4	3	32	39

Cakes, Pies, Puddings, Ice Creams & Cookies	*Protein*	*Fat*	*Carbo-hydrate*	*Calories*
Toast, plain 1 sl. 4″ x 4″ x ½″	8	2	40	50
Upsidedown cake 4″ x 3″ x 1½″	24	45	276	345
Vanilla wafers 4 of 2⅛″ diam.	8	27	68	103
Walnut wafers 1 of 2½″ x 3″ x 1″	4	72	64	140
White cake 2″ x 2″ x 2″	12	54	92	158
Zweiback 3 pcs. 3″ x 1½″ x ½″	12	18	68	98

Cheese	*Protein*	*Fat*	*Carbo-hydrate*	*Calories*
Brick 1″ x 2″ x ⅞″	44	135		179
Brie (American) 2½″ x 1¼″ x ¾″	40	99		139
Brie (French) 2″ x 2″ x ½″	36	126		162
Cheddar 1″ cube	20	54		74
Cream (Phila.) cheese 1 tbs.	12	63		75
Cottage (skim milk) 1 tbs.	11		3	14
Edam 1″ x 3″ x 1″	52	90	8	150
Grated 2 tbs.	8	27		35
Gorgonzola 1″ x 2″ x 1″	20	63		83
Gouda 1″ x 2″ x 1″	20	63	4	87
Gruyère 1″ x 4″ x ⅝	28	72	2	102
Liederkranz 1 tbs.	8	36		44
Limburger 3½″ x 4½″ x ½″	28	81		109
Münster 3½″ x 4½″ x ½″	24	81		105
Neufchatel 1 tbs.	4	54		58
New York 1″ cube	20	63		83
Parmesan 2 tbs. grated	16	27		43
Pimento processed 4″ x 4″ x ⅛″	16	54		70
Roquefort 1″ x 1″ x 1″	16	63		79
Soufflé, 1 c.	44	171	20	235

Cheese	Protein	Fat	Carbo-hydrate	Calories
Straws 3 of ⅜"	16	54	36	106
Stilton 1¼" x 3" x ¼"	28	90		118
Swiss American 4" x 4" x ⅛"	24	63		87
Swiss imported 4" x 4" x ⅛"	24	54		78
Tomato rarebit ½ c.	48	198	12	258
Velveeta 4" x 4" x ⅛"	16	45		61

Eggs	Protein	Fat	Carbo-hydrate	Calories
Duck egg 1	52	126	4	182
Goose egg 1	80	180	8	268
Hen egg 1	24	54		78
Omelet, French 1 egg	24	90	4	118
Omelet, plain 1 egg	28	81	4	113
Scrambled egg ½ c.	52	135		187
Turkey egg 1	80	162	12	254
Whites of egg 1	16			16
Yolks of eggs 2	20	90		110

Fats	Protein	Fat	Carbo-hydrate	Calories
Bacon fat 1 tbs.		99		99
Beef drippings 1 tbs.		99		99
Butter 1 tbs.		99		99
Butter peanut 1 tbs.	16	63	12	91
Cod liver oil 1 tbs.		99		99
Corn oil 1 tbs.		99		99
Cottonseed oil 1 tbs.		99		99
Crisco 1 tbs.		99		99
Halibut liver oil 1 tbs.		99		99
Lard 1 tbs.		99		99
Mineral oil 1 tbs.		99		99
Oleomargarine 1 tbs.		99		99
Olive oil 1 tbs.		99		99
Peanut oil 1 tbs.		99		99
Suet 1 c.	4	846		850

Fish	Protein	Fat	Carbo-hydrate	Calories
Abalone 2 of 4″ x 5″	112	117	12	241
Alewife 3″ x 2″ x 2″	88	27		115
Anchovies 3–4 fillets	8	9		17
Anchovy paste 1 tbs.	4	9	12	25
Barracuda, baked 3″ x 2″ x 1¾″	128	63		191
Black bass, baked 3″ x 3″ x 2″	116	135		251
Bonito, sautéed 3″ x 3″ x 1½″	160	108		268
Carp 3″ x 3″ x 1½″	84	27		111
Caviar, granular sturgeon tsp.	8	13		21
Caviar, pressed 1 tbs.	36	36		72
Clams, average raw 6 tbs.	24	9	8	41
Clams, canned meat, liq. ¼ c.	80	27	12	119
Clams, canned meat, liq. ¼ c. raw	16	9	4	29
Codfish balls 2 of 2″ diam.	32	126	44	202
Codfish, creamed ½ c.	48	63	32	143
Codfish, dry salt 4″ x 3″ x ¼″	116	9		125
Codfish, sautéed, fresh 3″ x 2″ x 2″	56	27		83
Crab, canned 1 c.	88	36	8	132
Crab, fresh 1 c.	84	18	4	106
Eels, smoked 2″ x 3″ x 3″	56	63		110
Finnan haddie 6 tbs.	44			44
Flounder ¾ c.	60			60
Haddock, smoked 3″ x 2″ x 1″	92	4		96
Halibut, broiled 4½″ x 3″ x ⅜″	88	54		142
Halibut, smoked 4″ x 2″ x ¾″	84	135		219
Herring, canned, tomato sauce 2 4″ x 1″ x 2″	64	90	16	170
Herring, kippered 1 of 4″ x 1″ x 2″	88	117		205

Fish	Protein	Fat	Carbo-hydrate	Calories
Herring, pickled Bismarck 1 of 4″ x 1″ x 1½″	80	135		215
Kingfish, baked 3″ x 3″ x 1″	96	108		204
Lobster, broiled 1 c.	80	18	4	102
Lobster, cocktail ½ c.	28	9	36	73
Lobster, canned 1 c.	92	18		110
Mackerel, sautéed 4″ x 3″ x 1″	104	162		266
Mussels, solids & liquid ½ c.	72	27	4	103
Oysters, canned 6 tbs.	24	9	16	49
Oysters, fresh	40	18	24	82
Oysters, fried 3 of 4″ x 2″	36	180	40	256
Perch, baked or broiled 3″ x 2″ x 2″	96	108		204
Perch, sautéed 1 whole	96	135	32	263
Pickerel, baked or broiled 3¼″ x 2″ x 2″	96	108		204
Red snapper, baked 3″ x ½″ x 4″	100	81		181
Roe, cod 4″ x 3½″ x ½″	48	9		57
Salmon, baked 5″ x 4″ x ½″	176	360		536
Salmon, canned ½ c.	104	99		203
Salmon, smoked 3″ x 2″ x 1″	88	81		169
Sardines, canned tomato sauce 2	80	81	4	165
Sardines, can oil	40	36		76
Scallops ½ c.	88		12	100
Scallops, escalloped ⅔ c.	80	144	52	276
Shrimp cocktail ⅓ c.	36	9	36	81
Shrimp, cooked or canned	24			24
Sole, baked or broiled 4″ x 2″ x ½″	88	45		133
Sole, sautéed 5″ x 2½″ x ⅝″	92	135	4	231
Sturgeon, smoked 2″ x 3″ x 1½″	124	18		142

Fish	Protein	Fat	Carbo-hydrate	Calories
Swordfish, broiled 3″ x 3″ x 1¼″	120	63		183
Trout, steamed	168	45	8	221
Tuna, canned	120	117		237
Whitefish, baked 2″ x 3″ x 2″	96	118		214

Flours	Protein	Fat	Carbo-hydrates	Calories
Bran, wheat ¼ c.	8	9	44	61
Buckwheat pancake flour 1 c.	64	27	392	483
Cornmeal, white 1 c.	48	45	384	477
Cornmeal, yellow 1 c.	48	45	384	477
Cornstarch 1 tbs.			36	36
Gluten flour 1 c.	236	27	268	531
Graham flour 1 c.	64	18	328	410
Oatmeal flour 1 c.	64	72	304	440
Pancake flour 1 c.	56	18	404	478
Potato flour 1 c.	48	9	448	505
Rice flour 1 c.	36	9	406	451
Rye, medium 1 c.	52	18	380	450
Soybean 1 c.	172	72	48	292
Wheat, cracked 1 c.	72	18	372	462
Wheat, whole 1 c.	68	27	376	471
Wheat, self-rising 1 c.	52	9	364	425

Fruits	Protein	Fat	Carbo-hydrate	Calories
Apple, average 1 of 3″ diam.	4	9	116	129
Apple, baked 1 large		18	244	262
Apple butter 1 tbs.			32	32
Applesauce, sweetened ½ c.			92	92
Applesauce, unsweetened ½ c.			52	52
Apricots, canned 4–7 & 3 tbs. juice	4		104	108

Fruits	Protein	Fat	Carbo-hydrate	Calories
Apricots, dried 5–6 halves	8		88	96
Apricots fresh 3–4	4		64	68
Avocado 1 medium	16	414	52	482
Banana 1 medium	4		80	84
Blueberries, fresh ¾ c.	4	9	76	89
Blackberries, fresh ¾ c.	8	9	60	77
Blackberries, canned, syrup ½ c.	4	9	76	89
Cherries, Maraschino 5			20	20
Cherries, sweet fresh 14–18	4	9	68	81
Cherries, sour 1 c.	4		52	56
Crabapples, fresh 1–2			16	16
Cranberries 1 c.	4	9	56	69
Currants, fresh 1 c.	8		52	60
Currants, dried 2 tbs.	4		76	80
Dates 2–3	4		60	64
Figs, canned 2 med.	4		60	64
Figs, dried 2–4	4		88	92
Figs, fresh 1 large	4		28	32
Gooseberries, fresh	4		52	56
Grapefruit ½ c. or 1 of 4″ diam.	4		44	48
Grapefruit, canned 1 c.	4		88	92
Grapes, American (Concord, Delaware) 1 bunch	4	9	60	73
Grapes, European (Malaga, Tokay) 1 bunch	4	9	132	145
Guavas, pineapple 1–2			36	36
Guavas, strawberry ½ c.	4		36	40
Kumquats 2–4	4		68	72
Lemons, fresh 1 of 2″ diam.	4	9	36	49
Limes, fresh 1–2			24	24
Loganberries, fresh ¾ c.	4	9	60	73
Loquats 6–8			32	32
Mangoes 2–3	4		44	48
Muskmelon ½ Large	4		48	52

Fruits	Protein	Fat	Carbo-hydrate	Calories
Muskmelon, cantaloupe ½ med.	4		36	40
Nectarines	4		64	68
Orange, fresh 1 of 4″ diam.	4		64	72
Orange, mandarin 1–2			20	20
Papaya, fresh 3″ wedge	4		40	44
Peach, fresh 1 med.			44	44
Pears, canned in juice 2 halves 2 tbs. juice			48	48
Pears, fresh 1 med.	4		64	68
Persimmon 1 med.	8	9	224	237
Pineapple, can 1 sl. or ½ c.			60	60
Pineapple, fresh ¾ c.			56	56
Plums, canned 2 med. 2 tbs. juice			80	80
Plums, fresh 1 large			20	20
Pomegranate 1 med.	4		96	100
Prunes, dried 6 small	4		100	104
Prunes, fresh 2–3 med.			20	20
Prunes, stewed 4–5 2 tbs. juice			80	80
Quince, fresh 1 large			112	112
Raisins, dried 2 tbs.			76	76
Raspberries, black 1 c.	8	18	80	106
Raspberries, red 1 c.	4	9	72	85
Rhubarb, fresh 1 c.	4		16	20
Strawberries, fresh 1 c.	4	9	40	53
Strawberries, canned juice ½ c.	4	9	40	53
Tangerines 4–5	4		44	48
Watermelon 1 sl. of 6″ diam.	4		40	44

Meat	Protein	Fat	Carbo-hydrate	Calories
Bacon, Canadian 4 sl. 2″ x 3″ x ⅛″	44	72		116
Bacon, crisp 4 sl. 2″ x 1½″ x ¹⁄₁₆″	24	126		150

Meat	*Protein*	*Fat*	*Carbo-hydrate*	*Calories*
Beef juice 1 c.	40	9		49
Bologna 2 sl. 2½″ diam. ⅛″	12	36		48
Brains, beef ½ c.	44	153		197
Chicken, broiler 1 med.	192	56		248
Chicken, canned ⅔ c.	240	144		384
Chicken, creamed ⅔ c.	76	342	20	438
Chicken, giblets ⅓ c.	92	56		148
Chicken pie 5″ arc x 3″ x 3″	164	162	132	458
Chicken, roasted 1 thigh or leg	112	72		184
Chili con carne ½ c.	72	27	186	285
Coney Island hot dog 1	44	135	64	243
Duck 3″ x 3″ x ¾″	128	45		173
Chuck, beef 4″ x 3½″ x 1″	96	162		258
Corned beef, canned 4″ x 3″ x ½″	100	108		208
Dried beef, creamed ⅞ c.	136	162	76	374
Dried beef ½ c. or 2 sl.	36	18		54
Flank, beef 2″ x 3″ x 2″	80	270		350
Frankfurter 1 of 3½″ length	24	72		96
Goose 3″ x 3″ x ¾″	88	63		151
Gravy, meat 3 tbs.	4	36	9	49
Hash ¾ c.	104	99	68	271
Headcheese 1 of 3″ x 4″ x 1/16″	20	54		74
Heart, beef 40″ x 3″ x ⅔″	108	54		162
Kidney, beef ½ c. or 2½″ x 2″ x 2″	124	108	8	240
Ham, boiled 1 sl. 4″ x 5″ x ⅛″	12	27		39
Ham, smoked baked 4″ x 2½″ x ¾″	112	171		283
Hamburger 1 of 3¼″ x 3″ x ¼″	36	108		144
Hash, corned beef ¾ c.	104	99	68	271
Lamb breast 4″ x 2½″ x 1″	140	405		545

Meat	*Protein*	*Fat*	*Carbo-hydrate*	*Calories*
Lamp chop, rib 1 of 4″ x 2″ x 1″	52	153		205
Lamb, leg of 3″ x 5″ x ¾″	120	135		255
Lamb chop, loin 1 of 4½″ x 3″ x ¾″	88	234		322
Lamb liver, or calf 5″ x 3″ x ⅜″	44	27	8	79
Liver, beef 5″ x 3″ x ⅜″	48	27	16	91
Luncheon meat 2 of 3″ x 4″ x 1/16″	20	72		92
Patty, 1 med.	108	270	72	450
Pâté de fois gras 1 tbs.	8	63	4	75
Pork chop	116	63		179
Pork chop, rib 3″ x 5″ x 1″	112	108		220
Pork feet, pickled ½ ft.	40	81		121
Pork loin roast 3″ x 4½″ x ¼″	120	90		210
Poultry dressing, bread ½ c.	16	63	88	167
Poultry dressing, rice wild ½ c.	44	81	172	297
Rabbit, domestic 1 leg 1 thigh	136	270		406
Rib roast, beef rare 4″ x 4″ x ¼″	76	171		247
Rib roast, well 4″ x 4″ x ¼″	104	135		239
Round, pot roast 3″ x 3″ x ½″	96	108		204
Round steak 3″ x 3″ x ¾″	96	108		204
Round steak, swiss 3″ x 3″ x ⅜″	96	135	68	299
Rump, beef medium 3½″ x 4″ x ½″	104	216		320
Salami 2 of 3″ diam. by 1/18″	24	81		105
Salt pork 3 sl. 2½″ x 1¼″ x ⅜″	32	252		284
Sausage, bulk 2 of 2″ x 1″	104	180		284

Meat	*Protein*	*Fat*	*Carbo-hydrate*	*Calories*
Sausage, link 3	32	81		113
Sausage, liver 2 of 2½″ diam. by ⅛″	12	27	16	55
Sausage, summer 3 of 1¾″ diam. by 1/16″	8	36		44
Side pork, fresh 6 of 2½″ x 1¼″ x 1/16″	92	27		119
Spareribs 2 of 5″ x 1½″ x 1½″	92	252		344
Steak, beef club, rare 3″ x 3″ x ½″	100	99		199
Steak, beef porterhouse rare 3″ x 3″ x ¾″	88	180		268
Steak, sirloin 4″ x 3″ x ½″ med.	80	117		197
Sweetbreads, veal ½ c.	88	36		124
Sweetbreads, med. fat ½ c.	48	324		372
Turkey 1 leg	116	171		287
Turkey, dark meat 4″ x 4″ x ¾″	160	45		205
Turkey, light meat 4″ x 4″ x ¾″	140	45		185
Tongue, canned or pickled 5 sl.	76	180		256
Tongue, beef 4 sl.	64	135		199
Veal chop, loin 1 of 3″ x 2½″ x ½″	92	54		146
Veal chop, rib 1 small	112	27		139
Veal kidney 1 whole	64	45		109

Milk	*Protein*	*Fat*	*Carbo-hydrate*	*Calories*
Buttermilk, cultured 1 c.	28	72	40	140
Buttermilk, plain 1 c.	28	9	37	74
Condensed milk ¾ c.	92	216	612	920
Cream, coffee ¼ c	8	108	8	124

Milk	Protein	Fat	Carbo-hydrate	Calories
Cream, heavy ¼ c.	4	189	8	201
Cream whipped 1 tbs.		27		27
Malted milk, choc. 1½ c.	44	162	200	406
Malted milk, plain 1½ c.	44	153	144	341
Milk skimmed 1 c.	28		40	68
Milk, whole 1 c.	28	72	40	140
Milk evaporated ⅔ c.	56	144	80	280
Milk, goat's 1 c.	28	72	40	140

Nuts	Protein	Fat	Carbo-hydrate	Calories
Almonds, choc. 10 med.	8	126	20	154
Almonds, plain 7	10	63	10	83
Almonds, salted 9–10	10	59	10	79
Butternuts 4–5	16	81	4	101
Brazil 6	16	180	12	208
Cashew 1 tbs. or 6–8	12	59	14	85
Chestnuts, dried 5–6	24	27	264	315
Chestnuts, fresh 6–7	4		68	72
Cocoanut, dried shredded ⅓ c.	4	81	64	149
Cocoanut, fresh 2 pc. 1″ x 1″ x ½″	4	90	16	110
Filberts 6–7	4	40	6	50
Hazelnuts ⅓ c.	8	36	64	108
Hickory 14–15 meats	8	90	8	106
Litchi 5–7			32	32
Nut, loaf ½ c.	18	90	44	152
Macadamia nuts ¼ c.	12	216	20	248
Peanuts, Spanish 2 tbs.	16	63	12	91
Virginia peanuts ½ c. or 12	24	81	20	125
Pecan nuts 6	4	90	8	102
Pine 3 tbs.	8	81	12	101
Walnuts, black 10–12 meats	12	81	12	105
Walnuts, English 10–12 meats	8	90	8	106

Sauces	Protein	Fat	Carbo-hydrate	Calories
Béchamel 2 tbs.	4	36	8	48
Butterscotch 2 tbs.		18	56	74
Caper 2 tbs.		4	27	31
Caramel nut ¼ c.		18	248	266
Cheese ½ c.		24	99	123
Cranberry 4 tbs.			152	152
Cream ½ c.	20	315	32	367
Curry ⅓ c.	28	54	28	110
Drawn butter ¼ c.	4	90	8	102
Egg 2 tbs.	12	54	12	78
English mushroom 2 tbs.		9		9
Fudge ¼ c.	4	82	288	374
Hard 2 tbs.		81	108	189
Hollandaise 2 tbs.	4	126		130
Hollandaise, mock 2 tbs.	8	54	12	74
Lemon 2 tbs.		18	40	58
Lemon with egg 2 tbs.	4	45	72	121
Maplenut ¼ c.	12	108	232	352
Marshmallow ¼ c.	4		108	112
Mint ¼ c.			20	20
Mustard 2 tbs.		27	4	31
Olive 2 tbs.	8	36	16	60
Orange 4 tbs.	4	45	44	93
Parsley 2 tbs.	8	45	12	64
Pineapple ¼ c.			200	200
Raisin 2 tbs.		9	88	97
Soy 2 tbs.	4		12	16
Tartar 1 tbs.	4	99	4	107
Tomato ½ c.	12	63	28	103
Vanilla ¼ c.		18	56	74
White ½ c.	20	144	36	200

Soups	Protein	Fat	Carbo-hydrate	Calories
Bean 1 c.	40	63	108	211
Bouillon 1 c.	8			8
Clam bisque ⅔ c.	12	27	24	63

Soups	Protein	Fat	Carbo-hydrate	Calories
Clam chowder 1 c.	42	153	88	283
Chicken ½ c.	16	9	12	37
Consomme ½ c.	24			24
Cream of asparagus 1 c.	36	127	64	227
Cream of celery 1 c.	16	126	64	206
Cream of corn 1 c.	40	126	140	306
Cream of mushroom 1 c.	28	126	52	206
Cream of pea 1 c.	47	126	100	273
Cream of tomato 1 c.	36	126	68	230
Lentil ⅔ c.	40	157	216	413
Oyster stew ⅔ c.	32	180	84	296
Potato 1 c.	24	36	100	160
Split pea ⅔ c.	28	36	68	132
Tomato, clear 1 c.	8		76	84
Vegetable ⅔ c.	8	18	36	62

Sweets, Sugars & Syrups	Protein	Fat	Carbo-hydrate	Calories
Butterscotch candy 5 of 1″ x 1″ x ¼″		9	72	81
Caramels 2 of 1″ cube	4	18	64	86
Caramels, choc. nut 2 of 1″ cube	4	45	56	105
Chocolate bar 1	60	459	36	555
Chocolate bitter, 1 square	8	135	20	163
Chocolate creams 2	4	36	72	112
Chocolate fudge 1″ x 1″ x 1″	4	27	92	123
Chocolate milk 3″ x 2½″ x ⅜″	16	162	104	282
Chocolate nougat 1″ x 1″ x ½″		18	68	84
Chocolate sweet 3½″ x 1½″ x ⅜″	4	135	20	159
Cocoanut creams ¾″ diam.	4	5	48	93
Dates, stuffed with nuts 2		9	56	65
Divinity 1¼ cube	4	18	84	106

Sweets, Sugars & Syrups	Protein	Fat	Carbo-hydrate	Calories
Figs, glacé 2–3 large	16		296	312
Frosting chocolate 5 tbs.	8	72	128	208
Gum drops 1 pc. of ½″ diam.	4		32	36
Hard candy ⅓ c.			396	396
Hershey bar, nut 1 small	24	163	76	263
Honey 1 tbs.			64	64
Jelly beans 9–10 large	8		168	174
Marshmallows ⅓ c. or 5	4		108	112
Mints, after-dinner 15 of ½″ square			176	176
Mints, cream 4–5			88	88
Molasses 1 tbs.	4		56	60
Nut bar 2″ x 3″ x 1⅛″	44	351	486	881
Peanut brittle 2 pc. 2″ x 2″ x ¼″	8	36	52	96
Peanut nougat 1″ x 2″ x 1″	16	45	40	101
Penuche 1½″ cube	4	18	80	102
Popcorn, plain 1 c.	4	9	48	61
Popcorn, with nuts 1 c.	20	81	248	349
Popcorn, sugared 1 c.	8	27	116	151
Praline, pecan 1 of 2″ x 3″ 1″	4	99	312	415
Stick candy 1 stick			52	52
Suckers 1			76	76
Taffy 2 cubes		9	76	85
Turkish delight 1½″ cube	4	18	84	106
Pears, glacé ½ large	4		304	308
Jam, strawberry 1 tbs.			64	64
Jelly (Heinz) 1 tbs.			64	64
Jelly grape 1 tbs.			52	52
Marmalade, orange 1 tbs.			68	68
Sugar, brown 1 tbs.			36	36
Sugar, corn 1 tbs.			60	60
Sugar, granulated 1 tbs.			60	60
Sugar, maple 1″ x 1½″ x 1″			180	180

Sweets, Sugars & Syrups	*Protein*	*Fat*	*Carbo-hydrate*	*Calories*
Sugar, powdered 1 tbs.			100	100
Syrup, corn 1 c.			888	888
Syrup, chocolate ⅓ c.	4	54	192	250
Syrup, maple 1 tbs.			52	52
Raspberry syrup ⅓ c.	4		160	164
Sorghum molasses 1 tbs.			52	52

Vegetables, Salads & Salad Dressings	*Protein*	*Fat*	*Carbo-hydrate*	*Calories*
Apricot & mayonnaise salad 1 serving	16	144	72	232
Artichoke ½ of 3″ diam.	12		48	60
Asparagus, canned 5–6 tips	4		8	12
Asparagus, french dressing salad 1 s.	4	81	12	97
Bamboo shoots ¼ c.	4		8	12
Beans, chili	12	18	60	90
Beans, kidney 7 tbs.	24		64	88
Beans, lima fresh ½ c.	32	9	96	137
Beans, lima dried ½ c.	80	9	248	337
Beans with pork 1 c.	52	45	172	269
Beans, string canned ½ c.	4		8	12
Beans, string fresh 6 tbs.	8		16	24
Beans, soy fresh ⅝ c.	54	63		117
Bean sprouts 1 c.	12		16	28
Beets, canned ½ c.	8		48	56
Beets, fresh ⅝ c.	4		20	24
Beet greens, fresh ½ c.	8		24	32
Beet Relish 2 tbs.	4		16	20
Broccoli 1 c.	16		28	44
Brussels sprouts 8 average	16	9	36	61
Cabbage, cooked ⅔ c.	4		12	16
Cabbage, raw 1 c.	4		20	24
Cabbage, Chinese	4		8	12
Carrots, cooked ½ c.	4		20	24
Carrots, raw 6 tbs.	4		20	24
Carrots, raw & mayonnaise	4	108	44	156

Cakes, Pies, Puddings, Ice Dressings	Protein	Fat	Carbo hydrate	Calories
Cauliflower ⅔ c.	8		20	28
Celery 2 Stalks	4		8	12
Celery root			8	8
Chard 1 c.	4		8	2
Cheese, pineapple, mayonnaise salad, 1 slice	8	171	52	231
Chicory ½ head	4		8	12
Chicken & mayonnaise ¾ c.	88	144	8	240
Chop suey, American ½ c.	40	216	12	268
Chow mein ¾ c.	20	143	24	187
Chutney 2 tbs.			96	96
Cole slaw (cream) 6 tbs.	4	27	20	51
Combination vegetable & french dressing	8	99	28	135
Cucumber ½ medium			8	8
Cucumber pickles sweet 1 small			28	28
Cucumber pickles sour or dill 1 large	4		8	12
Collards ½ c.	4		12	16
Corn, canned ½ c.	12	9	116	137
Corn, sweet fresh 1 ear large	20	18	120	158
Dandelion greens ¾ c.	16	9	56	81
Egg & mayonnaise salad	28	144		172
Eggplant 1 c. cubed	4		24	28
Enchilada 1 of 3″ x 5″ x 1″	56	180	156	392
Endive 4 to 5 leaves			4	4
Escarole 2 leaves			4	4
Fruit & mayonnaise salad ½ c.	4	99	44	147
Kale ½ c.	12	9	28	49
Kohlrabi ½ c.	8		28	36
Leek 1 of 5″	4		12	16
Lentils, dried 3 tbs.	40		100	140
Lettuce 2 to 3 leaves	—	—	—	—

Vegetables, Salads & Salad Dressings	Protein	Fat	Carbo-hydrate	Calories
Lettuce french dressing ½ head	8	72	8	88
Lima bean & french dressing ½ c.	4	72	44	120
Lobster salad & mayonnaise	32	117	12	161
Mushrooms, fresh	—	—	—	—
Mustard green ½ c.	12		20	32
Okra ¼ c.	4		16	20
Olives, green 4–5 medium	4	45	4	53
Olives, ripe 4–5 medium	4	63	4	71
Onion, dry 1 sm. or 3 tbs.	4		16	20
Onion, green 2 medium			8	8
Parsnips ¾ c.	8	9	94	111
Peas, canned ¾ c.	12		40	52
Peas, black-eyed ½ c.	92	9	248	349
Peas, creamed ½ c.	24	45	64	133
Peas, green ¾ c.	28		72	100
Pepper, green 1 of 4″ diam.	4		24	28
Pepper, red 1 of 4″	4	9	32	45
Pepper, stuffed with rice 1 large	36	198	168	402
Pineapple, cabbage & french dressing salad ½ c.	8	99	32	139
Potato chips 1 c.	8	81	48	137
Potatoes, french fried 4 pc.	4	27	40	71
Potato fried ½ c.	8	81	72	161
Potato, in skin 1 medium	8		92	100
Potato, mashed ½ c.	8	54	52	114
Potato & mayonnaise salad ½ c.	4	99	64	167
Potatoes, creamed ½ c.	12	63	60	135
Pumpkin, canned 3 tbs.			8	8
Sweet potatoes canned	8		124	132
Sweet potato ½ med. fresh	8		112	120
Radishes 4–5			8	8

Vegetables, Salads & Salad Dressings	Protein	Fat	Carbo-hydrate	Calories
Romaine ¼ head			4	4
Rutabagas ½ c.	4		28	32
Salsify ¾ c.	12	9	64	85
Sardine & french dressing salad 3–4 fish	44	90	12	146
Sauerkraut ¾ c.	4		20	24
Shrimp, peas & mayonnaise ½ c.	24	117	8	149
Spanish rice 7 tbs.	68	90	80	238
Spinach, canned ½ c.	8	9	12	29
Spinach, fresh 2 tbs. cooked or ¼ c. raw	4		4	8
Squash, summer ½ c.	4		16	20
Squash, winter ½ c.	8		40	48
Tamale pie 1 c.	140	135	84	359
Tomato, canned 1 c.	8	9	44	61
Tomato catsup 1 tbs.			20	20
Tomatoes, fresh 1 of 3" diam.	4		16	20
Tomato, cucumber & french dressing salad, 1 serving	4	72	12	88
Tomato, lettuce french dressing 1 serv.	4	72	16	92
Tuna and mayonnaise salad ½ c	60	117	4	181
Turnips ½ c.	4		16	20
Turnips, raw 1 med. or ½ c.	4		20	24
Waldorf & mayonnaise ⅔ c.	12	162	68	242
Yam 1 medium	16		164	180